Sylvia Wurm-Werner

Ashley Sapen

Emily Sapen

#WeAreSugar

Volume 1, No. 1

#WeAreSugar

The Young Life with Type 1 Diabetes

Strategies for a Life Without Limits

Sylvia Wurm-Werner

Ashley Sapen

Emily Sapen

Imprint:

Texts: © Copyright by Sylvia Wurm-Werner, Ashley Sapen, and Emily Sapen
Cover: Domenik Tews

TABLE OF CONTENTS

ABOUT THE AUTHORS	10
PREAMBLE	13
DISCLAIMER	16
CHAPTER 1	
TYPE 1, 2, 3 OR 4: WHICH DIABETES IS THIS ABOUT	18
COMMON CLICHÉS ABOUT DIABETES:	19
DIABETES MELLITUS TYPE 1: Juvenile	20
DIABETES MELLITUS TYPE 2: Adult-Onset	21
DIABETES MELLITUS TYPE 3: Hidden Diabetes	21
DIABETES MELLITUS TYPE 4: Gestational	22
OVERVIEW OF BLOOD SUGAR LEVELS	25
CONVERSION TABLE FOR BLOOD SUGARS	27

CHAPTER 2

DIABETES MELLITUS TYPE 1: THE DIAGNOSIS: WHO WERE WE? WHO ARE WE? WHO WILL WE BE?

STAGE 1: WHO WERE WE? VIVI'S, ASHLEY'S AND EMILY'S STORIES	30
TYPICAL SYMPTOMS OF TYPE 1 DIABETES	36
STAGE 2: WHO ARE WE?	38
TIPS IN DEALING WITH A NEWLY DIAGNOSED DIABETIC:	40
Stage 3: WHO WILL WE BE?	46
THE WISH BOARD:	49

CHAPTER 3

DIABETES: EDUCATION	52
PRIORITIZING DIABETIC TOPICS FOR ACCEPTANCE AND YOUR ENVIRONMENT	
HYPOGLYCEMIA	57
DIABETIC UTENSILS	63

THE BLOOD GLUCOSE TEST	64
EMERGENCY SITUATION	65
SAFETY BEGINS WITH SELF	68

CHAPTER 4

THE IMPORTANCE OF HEALTHY BREAKS	71
DEXCOM: A CONTINUOUS GLUCOSE MONITOR	76
THE SEVERELY HANDICAPPED PASS	78

CHAPTER 5

PARTY ON! - DIABETES & PARTIES	
ABOUT BASIC PROCUREMENT, DIPS AND PEE-BREAKS	83
DIABETES & ALCOHOL	85
OUR MASTERY STRATEGIES FOR PARTIES	88
DIABETES & DRUGS	94

CHAPTER 6

DIABETIC BUSINESS ETIQUETTE	96
TIPS OF A SUCCESSFUL DIABETIC	102

APPLICATION/INTERVIEW	
CONFERENCES & PRESENTATIONS	104
GOLDEN RULES	108

CHAPTER 7

EXPERIENCE WANDERLUST	111
DECISION MAKING	116
"HEALTH"	118
THE CHECKLIST	121
ENJOY A HOLIDAY	132
LONG TRIPS & FLIGHTS	139
TRAVELING WITH DIABETES: THE SHORT VERSION	142

CHAPTER 8

LIVING ALONE WITH DIABETES	147
DIABETES IN A RELATIONSHIP – AN OPEN WORD	153
CONFLICTS & HOUSEHOLD CHECK	159

CHAPTER 9

DIETARY CHANGE   165

CHAPTER 10

EXERCISING WITH T1D   180

CHAPTER 11

TYPE ONE DIABETES IN PREGNANCY   185

CHAPTER 12

INSULIN PUMP VERSUS PEN   197

CHAPTER 13

GROWING UP WITH T1D IN SCHOOL   213

CHAPTER 14

THE IMPORTANCE OF SUPPORT

SOCIAL MEDIA   221

DIABETES CAMP   222

CHAPTER 15

LAST WORDS OF ADVICE   224

GREATER THAN HIGHS AND LOWS	226
STAY INVOLVED	226
CLOSING WORD	228

We dedicate this book:

To our family: we could never thank you enough for all of the love and support you continuously provide,

Our friends: You keep us motivated to live a healthy, enjoyable, "normal" life just as all young adults should,

And to all of those who provide continuous support in our everyday lives, both in person and online.

ABOUT THE AUTHORS

Sylvia Wurm-Werner

Sylvia Wurm-Werner alias Vivi was diagnosed with type one diabetes in 2002. Although Vivi had wanted to become a pilot since childhood, the diagnosis caused an immediate discontinuation of this profession of interest. Many other professions are forbidden to diabetics.

It was this experience that drove her to "fight" the limits of diabetes imposed by others and find ways to lead a "life without limits".

After a dual study abroad of business and administration for several years, very challenging conditions then followed. Despite all adversities, she learned a lot about diabetes in various extreme situations.

Since June 2018 Vivi has been blogging on www.sugarbootcamp.com, Instagram, and Facebook about "Diabetes & Lifestyle": for a life without limits.

Ashley & Emily Sapen

Ashley and Emily Sapen are identical twin sisters. They were both diagnosed with type one diabetes in December 2003 at seven years old. Ashley was diagnosed first and was extremely brave. When she came home from the hospital, Emily was filled with nerves as she watched Ashley check her blood sugar and give her own injections. The twin sisters' parents realized Emily was also symptomatic after Ashley's first night back home. They packed their belongings and rushed back to the hospital, with Emily's diagnosis dating just three days after Ashley's.

Ashley and Emily were lucky that their diagnoses occurred throughout a holiday break from school. This gave at least a couple days for them and their parents to learn this new lifestyle and plan accordingly.

Although it was unfortunate to be labeled as having a chronic illness when returning to second grade, Ashley and Emily were blessed to have each other. Neither of them let this condition stop them from doing anything. They will share their experiences they have gained through growing up with type one diabetes throughout the following chapters. Their hard working and active lifestyles helped shape who they are today, as they started off with full-time careers in the medical profession.

It is not an easy journey living with type one diabetes; however they strongly believe the extra effort they put forth is necessary and also rewarding!

Ashley and Emily have been blogging their lifestyles daily on their combined @DoubleTheInsulin Instagram account and Facebook page. They inspire and help guide their followers on how to venture through life with type one diabetes without limits. The account is also used to educate the nondiabetic community on all aspects of type one. They connect with others through messaging and emailing to answer questions, offer support, and share their complex insight and experiences.

PREAMBLE

Vivi published her own original book in Munich, Germany, titled #iamsugar, strategies for a life without limits. This book is a sequel that will aim to share the strategies and knowledge of three experienced individuals living with type one diabetes, including insight particular to Germany and the United States.

This book is intended to give you and your surrounding environment a detailed introduction to the world of diabetes.

With the help of the compiled contents, you will be able to easily distinguish between the different topics. In this context, you will also familiarize yourself with blood sugar guidelines, tolerances, symptoms (such as hypoglycemia), and various counter-regulatory measures.

A household check is included, which will guide you to always have the most important tools on hand. In addition, the diabetic's environment is displayed as well as how others can best support newly diagnosed type 1 diabetics to avoid conflicts.

Furthermore, this book will provide skills on how to communicate your diabetes to the outside world and which strengths can be developed through the disease in your environment.

Information is included on how to find the most suitable profession as a type 1 diabetic. In addition, Vivi will show you how to begin and pursue a career with a chronic illness such as type 1 diabetes in all its ups and downs.

In this context, we also address sensitive issues, for example, applying for a disability card. Addressing such a topic may help you to make a decision and find where you can turn to apply for a card in order to keep your own efforts to a minimum.

Furthermore, the book provides you with all the details on traveling abroad with a chronic illness such as type 1 diabetes. Whether abroad short or long - the tips in this book will prepare you well for your travels.

Topics such as parties, alcohol and drugs, and diets are arranged and discussed in this book with helpful tips for you.

Finally, this book explains the preparations and course of a pregnancy with type 1 and provides you with a unique comparative analysis between the use of insulin pens and an insulin pump.

This book covers many basic life issues for young people with type 1 diabetes.

The Sapen sisters have added the following additional chapters to this sequel: Growing up as young children, T1D in grade school and college, the importance of support, and any advice in addition to Vivi's.

DISCLAIMER

The information in this book is based on our own experiences and does not serve as a substitute for professional diabetes counseling. Neither Vivi, Ashley, nor Emily are doctors; therefore, no therapeutic measures should be taken without first contacting a doctor or your healthcare provider who may influence your treatment decisions.

CHAPTER 1

TYPE 1, 2, 3 OR 4: WHICH DIABETES IS THIS ABOUT

According to The "International Federation Diabetes" in 2015, there are about 415 million diabetics worldwide. Estimates for 2040 predict an increase to 642 million people living with diabetes. The American Diabetes Association noted 30.3 million Americans living with diabetes in 2015.

There are about 1.25 million American children and adults that have type 1 diabetes. The German Diabetes Aid states that an estimated 6 million diabetics live in Germany, but only 10% of all diabetics correspond to the so-called "type 1" - colloquially also called "juvenile diabetes". Typically people between the ages of 0 and 35 suffer from this type of diabetes - that is, at a relatively young age. There is virtually only one common picture of diabetics anchored in the minds of society and the term is often generalized; therefore, it is not surprising that most of our fellow men neither know about nor can distinguish between several diabetic types.

This book focuses on type 1 diabetes. All topics that move and concern young people (and their first environment) after diagnosis are addressed here. In order to distinguish the so-called "Type 1" from the other types of diabetes, we will briefly discuss some clichés and significant differences between the types in this first chapter.

COMMON CLICHÉS ABOUT DIABETES:

- Only overweight people have diabetes.
- If a diabetic changes his diet and loses weight, he is healthy again.
- Diabetics are not allowed to eat sweets.
- Diabetics have to follow a specific diet.
- Most diabetics are old.
- Diabetes is inherited.
- Diabetics cannot have healthy children.
- All diabetics have to give injections.
- Diabetics get other illnesses more easily.
- Diabetics live a shorter life.
- Diabetics need insulin if they are low in sugar.

None of these statements are universal and applicable to all diabetics. The only thing that all types of diabetes mellitus have in common is a metabolic disorder with the common finding of hyperglycemia of the blood.

TYPE 1 DIABETES MELLITUS:
THE JUVENILE DIABETES

- Low genetic inheritability.
- Usually people of normal weight or (in the case of severe insulin deficiency) underweight people
- Type 1 diabetes is caused by a genetic predisposition that causes an organic autoimmune disease in which the pancreas stops working (destruction of beta cells).
- The production of insulin is completely stopped after the so-called "honeymoon phase" (absolute insulin deficiency).
- Diabetics have to regulate their food intake and metabolism with injections throughout their lives.
- Prevention of the disease is not yet possible.
- Most type 1 diabetics are diagnosed in childhood, adolescence, or early adulthood up to the age of 30.

TYPE 2 DIABETES MELLITUS:
THE ADULT-ONSET DIABETES

- High genetic inheritability.

- Most type 2 diabetics are older than 40 years. It is only since children have become severely and pathologically overweight that forms of type 2 diabetes can develop.

- Overweight or a predisposition to what is known as insulin resistance leads to the fact that although one's own insulin is still present in the body, it can no longer work properly (relative insulin deficiency).

- These patients can manage their diabetes by exercising more, eating differently, and losing the necessary amount of weight to decrease insulin resistance).

- The majority of type 2 diabetics are treated with medication via the form of pills.

TYPE 3 DIABETES MELLITUS:
THE HIDDEN DIABETES (HYBRID)

- Not always clearly identifiable.

- Causes can be:

    - Genetic defect

    - Disease of the pancreas

    - Hormonal disorders

- Metabolic diseases
- Infections such as rubella, etc.
- Treatment is determined by the degree of insulin deficiency.
- A reversible course of the disease is possible - in contrast to type 1.
- Type 3 often suffers from a special enzyme deficiency, which makes the utilization of nutrients more difficult.

TYPE 4 DIABETES MELLITUS: GESTATIONAL DIABETES

- On average, 9-12% of all pregnant women suffer from gestational diabetes.
- Possible causes:
    - Family or personal health history
    - Prediabetes & overweight
    - Most likely: inability to increase insulin secretion during pregnancy
    - Previous miscarriages
    - Previous pregnancy with birth weight over 4kg
    - Non-white race

- The treatment includes a strict diet and possible supplementary medication depending on the degree of severity.

- Gestational diabetes typically disappears after childbirth.

Comparing the Different Types:

In summary, it can be said that neither type 1 nor type 3 suffer from diabetes due to weight problems. They can neither prevent the disease nor get rid of it through a change in diet.

On the other hand, individuals with type 2 and type 4 diabetes mellitus have an increased BMI and a diabetic genetic predisposition can be the cause of the disease. These types can usually be prevented with a healthy and balanced diet.

With reference to the other clichés, all diabetics can eat normally - including sweets. However, they should consume these in moderation and adjust their medication (insulin dosage) accordingly. Good blood sugar control also enables normal fertility, the conception of healthy children, and a normal life expectancy.

Incidentally, it is incorrect for a diabetic to need insulin if he or she has low blood sugar.

Hyperglycemia and hypoglycemia are often confused in society.

The situation is different when there is too little sugar in the blood (non-diabetics also experience this from time to time). Here, with hypoglycemia, the affected person has to consume fast-acting carbohydrates in order to regulate the blood sugar again and to avoid fainting or coma.

If there is too much sugar in the blood, it is referred to as hyperglycemia. The body needs insulin to channel the sugar through the cells and break it down. Here insulin must be supplied to the body.

OVERVIEW OF BLOOD SUGAR LEVELS

Table 1: Blood sugars and normal values

	Normal Values (Fasting Glucose)	Oral Glucose Tolerance Test (2 hrs Post meal)	Hgb A1c
Normal	<100 mg/dl (6 mmol/l)	<140 mg/dl (<7.8 mmol/l)	<5.7%
Prediabetes	101-126 mg/dl (6.1-6.9 mmol/l)	140-199 mg/dl (7.8-11.1 mmol/l)	5.7-6.4%
Diabetes	>126 mg/dl (> 7 mmol/l)	>199 mg/dl (>11.1 mmol/l)	>6.5%

Table 2: Target values for diabetics

Time of measurement	mg/dl	mmol/l
After waking up and before meals (preprandial)	80-130 (optimal: below 110)	4-7 (optimal: below 6)
2 hours after meal (postprandial)	Below 180 (optimal: below 140)	Below 10 (optimal: below 7-8)
Before going to bed	90-150	5-8
HgA1c	<7% or estimated average glucose <154 mg/dL	< 8.6 mmol/l

Table 3: Conversion table for blood sugar values

mg/dl	mmol/l	mg/dl	mmol/l
40	2.2	250	13.9
50	2.8	260	14.4
60	3.3	270	15
70	3.9	280	15.6
80	4.4	290	16.1
90	5.0	300	16.6
100	5.5	310	17.2
110	6.1	320	17.8
120	6.7	330	18.3
130	7.2	340	18.9
140	7.8	350	19.4
150	8.3	360	20.0
160	8.9	370	20.6
170	9.4	380	21.1
180	10.0	390	21.7
190	10.5	400	22.2
200	11.1	410	27.8
210	11.7	420	23.3
220	12.2	430	23.9
230	12.8	440	24.4
240	13.3	450	25.0

As most people in the United States understand and use the mg/dl unit, the mmol/l value is widely used elsewhere to monitor BG levels. The previous table may be referenced to understand the comparison between the values.

Your "feel-good blood sugar values" can and should diverge marginally. In Vivi's experience, tolerable deviations are about 15%. When Ashley and Emily's blood sugars deviate outside of their "feel-good" range (about 80-140 mg/dl), they become symptomatic.

Discover your "feel-good values" with the help of many blood sugar controls and start by writing down your feelings as soon as you feel them. Ashley and Emily become aware of their feelings much quicker when the change in blood glucose is greater than 3mg/dL per minute.

Examples:

50 mg/dL = Hungry and shaking

100 mg/dL = Normal

180 mg/dL = Headache

200 mg/dL = Thirsty

220 mg/dL = Urinating frequently

300 mg/dL = Upset stomach, nauseous, etc.

Discuss these values with your doctor afterwards. Our life is not a table - so find out your reasonable, well-being values!

CHAPTER 2

DIABETES MELLITUS TYPE 1: THE DIAGNOSIS: WHO WERE WE? WHO ARE WE? WHO WILL WE BE?

STAGE 1: WHO WERE WE?

THE STORY OF 3 DIAGNOSES. VIVI'S DIAGNOSIS STORY IS FOLLOWED BY ASHLEY'S AND THEN EMILY'S STORY. EACH ARE UNIQUE, AS EVERY DIABETIC HAS THEIR OWN STORY.

Vivi's Story:

I remember it as if it were yesterday, but since then more than 15 years have contributed to my story. It was about June 2002. I was a 20 year old, normal weight, sporty and versatile young woman who wanted to be a pilot and see the world. Up to this point I could count on one hand when I had become ill with a flu or a cold. I would classify myself as being top fit - physically as well as psychologically.

I can no longer say exactly when which symptoms occurred, but I remember afterwards the most obvious ones that suddenly came upon me. For example, I never had the urge to drink much or often, but suddenly I had unimaginable thirst. I drank a 1 liter bottle and immediately afterwards I had the feeling to die of thirst again. My throat seemed to dry out and so I immediately got something to drink again - again and again. The weather was already warm at that time and I thought at first that my thirst was coming from the early summer heat. Sometimes I couldn't stand it anymore and ran to the sink to "drink the tap empty". Within one week my drinking behavior increased up to a water crate (12 bottles) within 24 hours.

An increased urge to urinate came from constantly drinking and again I slept no more nights right through. I no longer could sleep through the night. After a few days I was so exhausted that I could have fallen asleep everywhere. At the beginning I thought all this was a logical consequence.

P.S.: There were still no smartphones for research "in between"...

Suddenly my eyes worsened massively. When I didn't recognize my own father on the other side of the street, I began to seriously worry. A plausible connection between all these symptoms did not yet appear to me. This may also be due to the fact that I didn't know any diabetics at that time and had no points of contact at all with this disease.

After about two weeks, I finally went to my family doctor and told her what had happened. Basically I just wanted a an order to rest, because I was simply convinced that the symptoms were the result of pure exhaustion.

After a blood sugar test resulted over 270 mg/dl in my blood, I went directly to the hospital that same day. For a month, I went to the diabetic rehabilitation clinic in Bad Mergent-heim.

I had no idea that this would not only be the end of my flying dream, but also the way into a new life for me...

Ashley's Story:

As stated previously, I was seven years old when I was diagnosed in second grade. I remember specifically not feeling well in school. I cried in my seat in the afternoon school day for several consecutive weeks. The issue I struggled with was being unable to explain the way I was feeling; I just knew I felt "sick". It then became clear that these feelings occurred mostly after breakfast and lunch times. One night, my family was running errands after eating dinner out at a restaurant. I began crying because I felt "funny". Throughout the evening, my mother took several trips with me to the bathroom. The frequency and amount that I was urinating was unreal and my mom knew something was going on.

With my mom being a school nurse for over 25 years, she was concerned that the symptoms I was presenting with were parallel with those of diabetes. Unfortunately her suspicions were true. I was admitted to the hospital on Christmas Eve morning with an initial BG of 715 mg/dL and was diagnosed immediately with type one diabetes. I lived an active life as a seven year old girl, keeping busy with school and extracurricular activities. I was not quite old enough to understand the impact that this new diagnosis had on my life; however, my parents suddenly had to add diabetes into the mix of school, cheerleading, dance, swimming, soccer, daycare, and every other little thing that they managed in just one of their four children's lives.

On Christmas day, my parents and I were educated in my hospital room on the condition and steps we had to take. We were told this would be the new normal way of living life although I did not completely understand it at the time. I left the hospital the next day checking my own blood sugar and giving my own injections. Carbohydrates were something I learned along with the action of insulin and "ratios" to calculate insulin doses, but I could not thank my parents enough for their commitment early on and everything they have done for me.

Looking back now, my diagnosis couldn't have come at a better time. Being the age that I was and having the mindset I had, I stayed positive and developed good habits to take care of myself that I do not recall ever doing differently! I believe growing up around medical equipment, attending multiple appointments per year, and living the T1D lifestyle influenced my love for career of nursing.

Emily's Story:

While Ashley was in the hospital, my mother continuously thought and worried about my chance of being diagnosed with type one diabetes. She questioned all of the nurses, doctors, and educators that came in and out of the room and was reassured a number of times. She was told that in the case of one identical twin having T1D, there was a 1 in 2 chance of the other twin being diagnosed in his/her lifetime. Furthermore, the endocrinologist mentioned that the closest he had seen identical twins be diagnosed throughout his practice was 18 months.

The night following Ashley's arrival back home I slept in my parents' bedroom. After waking up three times throughout the night to use the bathroom, my mother decided to check my blood glucose in the morning. Her suspicions were confirmed with a blood sugar over 300 mg/dL and we packed up our bags for the hospital.

Other than presenting with polyuria- urinating frequently, I did not show any other signs at the time. When my height and weight were taken at the hospital, we discovered a weight loss of over five pounds since a previous check-up earlier that year. Weighing less than 50 lbs at seven years of age, it was pretty significant to lose more than 10% of my body weight.

I could not have imagined navigating through and learning about the new lifestyle without Ashley by my side. I remember hiding behind my parents and holding onto them tightly during annual check-ups as Ashley stood brave and received her vaccinations without even a flinch. Adding in all of the finger pokes and needles that come with type one diabetes, I felt so incredibly lucky to have Ashley's support right next to me.

TYPICAL SYMPTOMS OF TYPE 1 DIABETES:

- **Frequent urination:** In diabetes, the body tries to excrete the increased amount of sugar in the blood via the urine. Those affected therefore have an increased urge to urinate (polyuria).
- **Strong thirst:** An increased urge to urinate can result in a lack of water. People affected then feel an increased need to drink.
- **Dry or itchy skin:** Dry skin can be a first sign of diabetes. It also occurs when the body excretes more sugar through the urine and loses fluid.
- **Fatigue:** An elevated blood sugar level often makes people feel listless.
- **Weight Loss:** In some cases, diabetes leads to weight loss. One reason for weight loss is due to the loss of fluid as a result of the increased urge to urinate. Another possible cause is that the cells are no longer able to sufficiently cover their energy requirements. This is due to elevated blood sugar levels causing the inability of sugar to reach the inside of each cell; therefore, the body falls back on fat deposits.
- **Wounds heal worse:** In diabetes, the immune system is often weakened. This factor and substandard blood circulation in the skin contribute to the slower healing of

wounds.
- **Increased susceptibility to infections:** Increased blood sugar levels burden the immune system. Diabetics are therefore more susceptible to various infectious diseases, such as athlete's foot, urinary tract infections, colds, yeast infections, and flu infections. Periodontitis also occurs more frequently in diabetes.
- **Acetone smelling breath**: Only with type 1 diabetes can an acetone smell become noticeable in the breath, which can be a similar odor of overripe fruit. If there is not enough sugar in the cells, the body breaks down fat cells. This produces acetone, among other things. It is a sign of a severe insulin deficiency, which can lead to ketoacidosis and in the worst case to diabetic coma and death.

STAGE 2: WHO ARE WE?

If I, Vivi, had been told beforehand that I would have to inject myself for the rest of my life, I probably would have replied that I would rather die. Everything changes when you suddenly have the certainty that you will die without the injection!

During the insulin adjustment in the hospital I suffered terribly from the constant and regular blood tests, because syringes and I did not get along. In the morning, at noon, and in the evenings, blood was taken from me, stress tests were carried out, carbohydrate measurements were made , insulin injections were dosed and injected, and so on.

Efforts were made to determine how many units of insulin I needed for the carbohydrates I consumed and how my body processes them throughout various activities.

The nurses kept bouncing around ideas about how quickly one would get used to it....

Today I know they were conditionally right! You get used to measuring blood sugars and carbohydrates and injecting insulin after a while. Everything else that belongs to this disease - the constant stress change that is simply part of life -

remains a constant battle with diabetes, but above all, with yourself.

To "ram" the syringe into your stomach for the first time is incredibly difficult. One is first overwhelmed by irrational fear of it. In the beginning you don't know the right places and grips on your body or the most painless degree of puncture. You just don't have a fine-tuning feeling yet. If one realizes shortly after that this is now a forever vital for one, one experiences pure despair.

With me and others. I have experienced and understood the following phases in my illness:

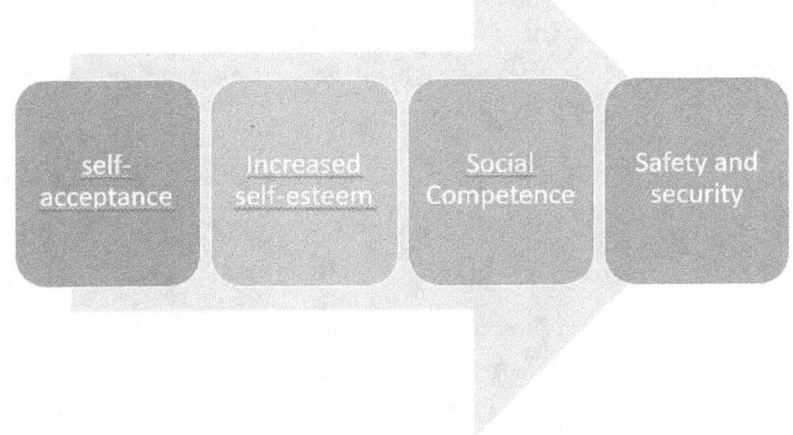

Comments from friends and relatives who try to trivialize the illness of the affected person during the "realization and acceptance process" in order to offer comfort should be held back with their "well-intentioned comments", because it can in turn have a negative or aggressive affect on the individual.

- Consider the four phases presented above and acknowledge that no one - except for the person concerned himself - knows what it feels like and what task he is facing. The only exception to this may be when siblings are diagnosed within a short time period and are adjusting to this new lifestyle together, facing new challenges at the same time. Neither during the diagnosis nor in the further course of the disease do diabetics need commentary on the disease or how it is handled by our healthy environment.

TIPS IN DEALING WITH A NEWLY DIAGNOSED DIABETIC:

- Are you interested in nutrition? Try "diabetic food" in cooking and baking - you will notice that it is nothing else than a balanced and healthy diet. This requires less change than some allergy sufferers and the type of diet is good for everyone - and even trendy!

- If you are not the "cooking type", but would like to offer a useful present to the person concerned, then buy him/her a great cookbook. Cookbooks from "Weight Watchers" or the "Paleo Diet" are well suited for diabetics and are very inspiring and delicious.
- Instead of commenting or saying "comforting words", behave normally and give the affected person the feeling of maintaining normality in everyday life with your support.
- Refrain from voicing suggestive sentences, questions, or judgments that express disapproval or disappointment such as "what if...", "perhaps you would have...", "others have it better under control because..."...

  A type 1 diabetic cannot do anything for his illness and could have neither prevented nor averted it.

- Furthermore, the affected person must always control his illness similar to handling a car - over stick and over stone, day and night. Sometimes the "car" drives smoothly around curves, sometimes it comes to a standstill or has a breakdown... It may be that the breakdown is "due to holes in the road" or was caused by your own "driving style".... Since you, as a relative, cannot drive this "car", please do not be a "backseat driver".

Before you question the "way of driving", it is better to offer help to repair the "breakdown" - even if you are simply there with a personally addressed request to "tackle" and wait together with patience, until the "car" drives on again...

- Ask questions that express your interest in diabetes and say that you are dealing with the disease in the same way and will not leave the person affected alone in dealing with diabetes.

- Support the sick person during his hospital and rehabilitation stay by looking for a good diabetologist (endocrinologist or diabetes educator) and making a well-founded recommendation to the affected person.

  If you are interested, talk to endocrinologists, pharmacies, the health insurance company or the Red Cross etc. and let them prepare you for what you will have to do as a relative - or what role you can play.

- Examples of topics to become knowledgeable on include: symptoms of hypoglycemia, what an emergency appears like, and how to prepare and administer the emergency medication (glucagon).

- Are there diabetes trainings offered in your

area? The affected person must attend such training during hospitalization, rehabilitation, and/or afterwards. There are also training courses which relatives can/should attend - it is now even welcomed by health insurance companies! Inform yourself and if you are interested and try to participate in such a course.

- From now on, store glucose in all your bags or drawers and always have a juice in the fridge!

  In the beginning, the diabetic himself is not always organized and does not have the experience to know what is necessary. One might unintentionally be without aids or extra sugar outside the house. It is comforting to a diabetic when they realize a loved one has thought for them in an emergency and thus averts a "dicey" situation.

- If the person concerned is still a child or adolescent, seek a discussion with responsible persons such as teachers, sports coaches, or parents of child friends.

- In Germany, the social association VDK also represents the interests of disabled people and handles the application for severely disabled cards. Collect information about this which could be of help to the person concerned.

It is a sensitive issue for people with disabilities - I (Vivi) did not want to apply for an ID card for more than 10 years for (false) pride. However I was also not aware of the various advantages, such as tax savings and many benefits in everyday life.

Here is a link we found in which you can learn more about the provided benefits and opportunities for life and work for those able to receive the card:

www.angloinfo.com/how-to/germany/healthcare/people-with-disabilities/disability-benefits.

There is not yet something such as this that exists in America. Further information can be found in a later chapter (Chapter 4).

- Perhaps you and the endocrinologist would like to summarize the most important information together and write down emergency telephone numbers. Distribute this "leaflet" to all people necessary. It is a good idea to educate and sensitize the parents of the child's friends who will interact with your diabetic child. They could draw their children's attention to certain symptoms to possibly notice something may be occuring.

- In the case of young diabetics, it is better to discuss a common approach.

Adolescents already have many arguments with themselves, feel quickly patronized, and sometimes like to block such things from their parents. That would be fatal here!

Type 1 diabetes mellitus is a serious disease; however, your adolescent child should not have the feeling that they are being deprived of their own freedom or "the air to breathe". They should rather understand what diabetes means and what they should pay attention to on their own.

Offer yourself as a parental supporter - but don't impose. Your adolescent child should first get a chance from you to prove how adult he or she can handle this diagnosis.

STAGE 3: WHO WILL WE BE?

Even as a young person it is hard to be able to say goodbye to goals, dreams, and desires, or to be able to reflect on your peers without hesitation or reflection. For example, Vivi once wanted to become a pilot. Unfortunately for her, the diagnosis "type 1 diabetes" meant the dream of flying was over faster than it had begun. On the search for vocational alternatives, she noticed that one with type 1 Diabetes may exercise no occupation in which one has responsibility for other human lives. In addition, occupations where one cannot briefly interrupt its activity to control and regulate the sugar are also prohibited. Such professions include bus drivers, train drivers, tram drivers, pilots, air traffic controllers, professional divers, and even policemen.

Despite today's revolutionary treatment methods, most employers and companies see a great risk that a clouding of consciousness could occur as a result of hypoglycemia. After all, police officers carry weapons and drive vehicles with special signals through traffic.

If one learns of his professional limitations as a type 1 diabetic, it is of course useless to stick one's head in the sand -although this is usually the first measure everyone likely takes. One feels disadvantaged, unfairly treated and judged, and sees and feels the risk differently than outsiders.

What remains are certain abilities and potentials that diabetes cannot take away! The next step is to analyze them and rearrange your "old wishes" in order to come close to them with a different job profile. Basically it is nothing else than to set yourself a new goal and to replace and say goodbye to the other.

We are thankful that in the U.S. we have not been limited in occupational opportunities due to our condition, or at least since the time we began searching for our choice of jobs. It may be different now than Vivi's explained experience, but it is certainly important to research what you have a passion for and if your choice of career path is possible.

THE TALENT should determine the career choice - not our diabetes!

In Vivi's case, she first had to deal intensively with herself, rethink, and reschedule what she personally wanted to do and achieve in life.

Never forget your ideas right away. Give them a realistic chance of success. Think about how you could successfully implement your ideas, how much effort this will mean, how much time it can (and may) cost, and whether it is enjoyable. Don't ask yourself if your diabetes is hindering an idea. Ask yourself HOW you can integrate your diabetes and find a suitable, integrative way!

My (Vivi's) approach had become more systematic over the years through using the method of self-image and external image analysis to organize her skills and interests. In the course of this analysis, I have looked at models - people I admire. I take a closer look at their job descriptions and related professions. I write down in keywords what my idea of them is and read through the corresponding job advertisements. In between, I compare these with my abilities in a renewed self-image and external image analysis. Just because I find something great - e.g. acting - doesn't mean that I have the skills and the tools to do the job. Even if I had the talent to be an actor, I would have to question whether I could live - if successful - with my "fans" wanting to know everything about me, paparazzi chasing me and no secret remaining undiscovered...

I'm also thinking about what I have to earn to finance my life. This includes what I want to earn and what I want for my life...

The subject is very complex. But since it will shape your future, it is really worthwhile to "sacrifice" time for this, to reflect and to discuss with people who are close to you.

If you do not find the help you need in your environment or if you need support, I recommend my online coaching. One example to search for a suitable career is below:

THE WISH BOARD:

Get a pin board, a magnetic board, or a notepad. Start a brainstorming session with yourself - and possibly someone you trust. What special skills do you have?

What hobbies do you have or have you always wanted to develop?

Do you think about which activities are better than average for you and whether you enjoy it?

What do you dream of in life? (Fame, money, family, a house? Do you want to live abroad, in the country or in the city? etc.)

<u>Now, you deal with it as it follows:</u>

- Write everything down in keywords.
- Search for images (on the Internet, for example) that visualize these keywords.
- Prioritize the keywords & images.

- Cluster them: Which of your abilities, hobbies & wishes can be summarized or exercised together?
- Now name it.

Which job profiles suit this idea?

In the beginning, you may spontaneously have no idea which job title fits your abilities and wishes. That's why you hang all the pictures you've selected for the keywords and summarized them in a "cluster" on your pin wall. For example, you may be very creative in one of your "clusters": you like to paint privately, abstract thinking distinguishes you from the average, you dream of a free life, want to live in nature, like to live in a house and sometime with a family.

It can be that after only one day "a light comes on" or it takes a week, a month, or longer. It is important that you have structured and visualized your thoughts. Every time you now look at your pinboard - your wish board - you will notice something and you will automatically focus on it.

In other words, it helps you to focus on and deal with your ideas and wishes, from which concrete goals can emerge at some point and a path can (and will!) grow.

Maybe you're redoing certain things or changing your priorities afterwards. Whatever you do - every time you look at the board of your choice, you come closer to your implementation and your goal.

If you come across some job titles, search for suitable "job descriptions" on the Internet. If you don't find a job description, look for advice from someone - such as the employment agency.

With various "job descriptions" you are now one concrete step further. Evaluate the different job requirements against your abilities with school grades. Grade 1 can stand for "I can do very well" and grade 6 for "I can't do anything". Then calculate an "average grade".

Hang up the prioritized job list on your wish board. Now you should slowly develop a gut feeling which job suits you best and your abilities and dreams!

CHAPTER 3

DIABETES-EDUCATION - HOW TO SAY IT IN SCHOOL / EDUCATION / STUDY / JOB?

Don't exaggerate, just say enough.

If there's one thing we have all learned in recent years, it's that it is beneficial and not embarrassing to have as many people as possible know about yourself and your diabetes. Of course, you don't want to (and shouldn't) keep talking about your diabetes or confront people with the "ups and downs" (our blood sugar levels) because they can't possibly understand.

It also doesn't get you into the details to ramble about medications, dosages, injecting techniques, or readings (literature/research).

Most of our fellow humans react quickly bored with too much information or directly distance themselves due to disgust in connection with blood, syringes, and so on. That is unless you happen to work in the medical field and are educating curious coworkers!

It is a gradual hike for us affected people to inform as many people as possible in our environment about our illness and to sensitize them without being immediately labeled as ill, ignored, or "specially" treated.

Here are our tips:

The communication of our diabetes should be preceded by a precise objective and consequently we must use our empathy carefully, accurately, and methodically. Strictly speaking, it is about "placing our story" in time in bite-size bits of information to be effective. If you can instinctively arouse curiosity and interest in your surroundings, you will avoid immediate negative feelings such as pity or even disgust.

- In this way we can use our communication to reveal and communicate important information about our disease that is understood and taken into account in a sustainable way.

- It is difficult to learn empathy because it is something we all carry within us - sometimes stronger and sometimes weaker.

- In addition, empathy strength also depends on our own self-perception. It is the ability to recognize and understand the thoughts, emotions, motives and personality traits of another person. This is necessary in order to successfully control the aforementioned communication of our disease.

- First of all, sit down with the advantages that arise when as many people as possible in your environment know about your diabetes.

- **Safety**

    If your environment knows about possible diabetic risks and symptoms such as low blood sugar and what to do in case of an emergency, you will gain protection if you are not feeling well or possibly even lose consciousness.

- **Respect & Consideration**

    If you bring your illness across "strongly", you will be paid in respect for all your activities and efforts, such as your working pace, your overtime efforts, or other "special" achievements.

    If you earn praise for being "normal", you will at the same time gain more consideration if you are feeling down on weak days and must take it slowly, have to go to an extra doctor's visit, etc.

- **Tolerance & Acceptance**

    You may need an extra break because you have to measure your blood sugar, go to the bathroom more often, or periodically struggle with hyperglycemia or hypoglycemia.

    Or have you ever forgotten your glucometer and had to drive back home, making you late for appointments or work?

If people know about your illness and the hurdles associated with it, you will usually be looked at with tolerance and acceptance in exceptional situations.

As you may have noticed, I increasingly speak of "strengths" in the execution of possible advantages. One of my basic rules - which is also the basis for successful communication - says:

Never let your diabetes bring you down and always make yourself comparable with "healthy" colleagues or friends and family members - despite occasional "handicaps".

Are you now thinking carefully about who you like to listen to and alternatively slightly admire yourself?

- Is it the plaintive patient?
- Or are they the ones who make the most of your illness, perhaps even develop special skills such as "foot painting" when they no longer have arms?
- Are they monotonous and full of self-pity, always telling the same dramatic stories, cruel experiences, and sad life events?
- Or are they rather those who, alone with their ability to tell, cast a spell over you - whether funny, exciting, theatrical, sarcastic, parodic, or

critical?

- Or a special narrative style - without mourning or depression in the voice, which stands out from the majority and always wins listeners.... no matter what kind of story is being told.

This strong, narrative ability separates itself from any monotonism and self-pity and radiates strength and self-confidence. Characteristics that magically attract fellow human beings. Influential people are and always will be good speakers, who inspire the thinking of their listeners even if they are not particularly interested in the topic to be presented. If words convey a certain commitment and confidence, you begin to inspire your fellow men- and to communicate your diabetes with it, subliminally and effectively, positions you to coach your uneducated and inexperienced environment.

Do you wish to compile your story effectively and are unsure how it really works? Vivi's' online coaching program includes creating your communication guideline with the help of an individual storyboard. Ashley and Emily are also available to discuss this with you via their Instagram and Facebook page!

PRIORITIZING DIABETIC TOPICS FOR YOUR ENVIRONMENT

HYPOGLYCEMIA

It is beyond question that the most important topic in communication is first and foremost dealing with hypoglycemia. All other topics, one can scatter with interest gradually, but hypoglycemia happens frequently and represents an everyday challenge for type 1 diabetics.

Signs of hypoglycemia?

Sweating, dizziness, tremors, lack of concentration, blurred vision, palpitations, cravings, dilated pupils, headaches.

What does the diabetic need during a hypoglycemic episode?

Fast-acting carbohydrates = sugar that goes quickly into the bloodstream, e.g.:

- o Dextrose (in the form of glucose tablets, candy, liquid, powder)
- o A banana or fresh grapes
- o Juice (apple or grape juice work well)
- o Lemonade, Coke, or other regular soft drinks
- o Gummy bears...etc.

In an emergency situation, it is extremely important to decide in seconds whether you first have to measure your blood sugar or go straight to ingesting some form of sugar.

Doctors/healthcare providers would generally recommend that you first check your BG and then consume a specific amount of fast-acting carbohydrates in a controlled manner. As diabetics for many years, we are accustomed to carefully disagree at times with the general recommendation.

As a diabetic you normally feel whether the hypoglycemia is severe or mild. If you are still feeling under control and are only experiencing mild symptoms, then follow the typical advice and first check your blood sugar.

If you are experiencing hypoglycemia and your symptoms match a glucose somewhere below 70 mg/dL we may deviate from testing for the result first. It is vital to take a controlled intake of 15 to 30 grams of fast-acting carbohydrates. If you are certain that your BG is low or falling quickly, treat yourself first because it is a lifesaving measure. Then check your glucose. We have learned that generally 4g of glucose raises one's sugar about 10-15 points. I (Vivi) think: if one is overcoming a hypoglycemic state and is able to work but is active, one may want to ingest closer to 20-25 grams of carbohydrates to reach stability and feel well enough to work (a range from 100-120 mg/dL). If the BG reading is below 50 mg/dl, one may take about 30 fast acting carbohydrates and recheck the BG approximately every 15 minutes to test whether the added sugar was sufficient. It is important that you allow yourself a short rest in such hypoglycemic phases. Sit or lie down somewhere until it raises to a normal level.

With the use of modern technology such as continuous glucose monitoring systems, it is a bit easier to catch hypoglycemia. Low blood sugar is not completely avoidable and the diabetic must completely understand how to treat hypoglycemia before in extreme danger .

If an individual is always in motion and busy onto the next activity, he may have the tendency to consume a surplus of carbohydrates. The extent of continuous activity may give the individual a feeling that the typical 15 grams of carbohydrates is not enough to raise the BG. An important practice for a diabetic to abide by is to avoid "over-treating" a low blood sugar. The hungry and shaky feeling may cause one to "eat everything in sight". Try to adhere to the basics: treat with 15 grams and recheck in 15 minutes to reevaluate the situation.

From experience, the twins have found it difficult to limit sugar at times while on the go at work, running errands, or wanting to sleep, etc. Vivi has also experienced the inability to consume a controlled amount of carbohydrates due to a severely low BG. She only stopped eating when she noticed that her sugar was rising again and that she was out of danger.

The danger here is that you slip from a very deep sugar into a dramatically high sugar, otherwise known as rebounding. One my end up "chasing their tail" the rest of the day through over-treating a low BG, increasing insulin to bring the glucose down, falling low again, and repeating.

It has already happened that I (Vivi) slipped further into a hypoglycemia after injecting too much insulin, despite an intake of 40 grams of carbohydrates. By constantly measuring the course of the disease through glucose monitoring and adding more carbohydrates as needed, I was still able to protect myself from unconsciousness.

If one does not take time to rest the body, he will overexert himself too quickly and simply run into a hypoglycemic state again. We cannot reiterate enough how vital it is to control the sugar intake and rest the body to heal itself of hypoglycemia. When one will be jumping right back into strenuous activity, treating first with fast-acting carbohydrates and then a bit of protein/fat will help the sugar to level out and stay stable rather than spike downward again.

In some instances, urgency takes precedence over protocol. With experience comes techniques to treat your BG in different instances. Also, every diabetic reacts to glucose a little differently. Some people may need very little to correct a hypoglycemia (e.g. only 10 grams of carbohydrates), whereas it may take others 30 minutes or more to recover from the same blood sugar.

Vivi's motto stands: **It is better to end up with a controllable and predictable hyperglycemia than the risk of dying from massive hypoglycemia.**

Ashley and Emily also believe in this motto. Although the length of time of high blood sugar levels should be as brief as possible to minimize long-term complications, it is not as urgent and life-threatening as a low blood sugar.

A piece of advice:

If you suddenly become symptomatic with hypoglycemia or hyperglycemia while traveling alone, for example on a public bus, be sure to do the following:

Jot down all important data::

- Time
- Blood sugar value
- Your action (sugar intake or correction)

Perhaps you carry a blood sugar diary with you at all times. If not, it is a decent idea to have a pen and notepad on hand or even a charged cellular device in which you can leave a note on.

If you should pass out, passengers or first-aiders can quickly determine what is going on with you on the basis of the note or your diary. As long as you have control over yourself, look around to see if you can find someone who seems trustworthy to you. If your fear unconsciousness or the thought of it increases, approach that person and speak to them. Let the stranger know that you are a type 1 diabetic, the current situation, whether the lady or gentleman would be so kind to stay with you until you feel better and, if necessary, make an emergency call.

Sometimes the single idea of having someone close by can help. It is also reassuring if you have all the important data in your hand and document it (through a blood sugar diary), because you will always contribute to your first aid if it is necessary.

DIABETIC UTENSILS

We recommend to carry all "diabetes utensils" in a recognizable bag.

For example, Vivi has her diabetes equipment in a bag with cat pictures on it. In her environment everyone knows the term "cat bag" and knows that it means the bag containing all of her essential diabetes utensils.

Ashley and Emily enjoy searching for fashionable wristlets (MySugarCase being one) that fit their frequently used supplies in throughout the day. Just as important, they both carry small bags/sacks that are designated for their "extra and emergency supplies". These can fit in a work bag and purse to be prepared for the time when new test strips, a vial of insulin, a new insulin pump site, batteries, syringes, glucagon, etc. is needed. It happens more often than you can imagine

In cases of panic, it helps your surrounding environment to search for and find them. Since many are not familiar with what an insulin pen or blood glucometer looks like, it is necessary to support your fellow human beings by carrying your essentials in a bag that can be briefly and concisely described.

THE BLOOD GLUCOSE TEST

Many healthy people around us find blood sugar testing exciting and would also like to know how high or low their level is. Always use a fresh lancet for this.

When measuring, the blood comes into contact with the lancet, which is why each user should use their own lancet. If someone around you wants to know his or her blood sugar, others may quickly come along and suddenly there is a whole group around you.

Do not forget at this moment that you may only receive a limited number of BG test strips each quarter of the year and that these are very expensive at about 50 cents/strip. If you are reaching near the end of your supply on hand, be courageous and honest enough to refuse your fellow human beings the wish to measure their BG or be a charming liar and use the missing, fresh lancet as an excuse.

EMERGENCY SITUATION

When learning in the initial diabetic training courses, it is taught that type 1 diabetics should always carry a glucagon injection kit with them. According to expert opinion, this is included in the standard equipment of a diabetic. The glucagon is a "rescue glucose medication" and is best injected into the thigh if you are dangerously hypoglycemic or even unconscious. This life-saving injection acts in this way: glucagon allows the glycogen stored in one's liver to be released and be converted into glucose, being immediately delivered into the bloodstream. This mechanism results in a rapid elevation of BG within minutes.

Consider this: The glucagon injection must be administered by another individual when the diabetic is in a state of severe hypoglycemia. The diabetic may be presenting with a decreased level of consciousness, lethargy, or seizure activity. With this being said, the following must also be considered:

- a natural fear of syringes. The vast majority of our fellow human beings do not come from medical professions or have experience with injections.
- Furthermore, in the case of unconsciousness, the observing person may not instinctively know whether it is due to hypoglycemia or

hyperglycemia.

- If Glucagon is injected in the case of hyperglycemia, this measure can unfortunately further worsen the issue or lead directly to exitus in extreme situations. However, if our fellow helper waits too long and first tries to determine the diabetic's blood sugar laboriously (because untrained), vital time is lost. Instead time would be better invested with a call to the emergency doctor.

- Almost none of us surround ourselves with the same people every minute of the day. It is practically impossible to teach everyone how to use a glucagon syringe.

It is important to make sure that your environment is aware of your diabetes. A simple and sufficient plan would be to have them call your emergency physician (or 911) immediately and briefly describe to them the recognizable symptoms and actions leading up to the emergency.

Teach your family, friends, close coworkers, and medically trained friends how to prepare and use the glucagon. Review it with them periodically because emergency situations typically do not run as smooth as the review process. Believe it or not, a cell phone application exists in which individuals can virtually practice glucagon preparation and administration. Ashley and Emily's friends and family have had the benefit of practicing the emergency procedure hands-on with expired Glucagon kits. The Sapen twins would first demonstrate the process and then the individual performed the procedure back, injecting the solution into an orange or telephone book.

Additional tips:

It is best to carry a clearly visible diabetic ID card in a spot easily accessible- for example in your wallet or a clearly defined medic-alert bracelet. Meanwhile, there are also very modern alternatives such as diabetes tattoos, bracelets, necklaces, ribbons, as well as accessories for smartwatches and phones.

When the witness is calling 911 or the emergency doctor, the individual does not need to have a medical background or have a complete understanding about type one. The trained professional is proficient in testing a glucose level, understanding symptoms and risk factors, and will decide accordingly whether to instruct to administer glucagon or insulin.

In summary, we recommend the diabetic to inform their daily environment on the following topics:

- Hypoglycemia and its symptoms
- Appropriate measures to treat hypoglycemia (supply of sugar)
- Storage of your medical equipment (possibly also your sugar diary)
- Use of the glucometer and understanding the sugar values
- Persons to be notified in an emergency (doctor, relatives)
- Use of the glucagon syringe

SAFETY BEGINS WITH SELF-ACCEPTANCE

Time and time again, we have discovered that a lot of things arise by themselves and develop positively with acceptance of oneself or a situation.

After I (Vivi) had finally accepted diabetes as part of myself, I stopped feeling ashamed to measure my blood sugar and inject insulin in public. My environment still reacts with interest and admiration about my self-confident handling of the lifelong condition. That helped me to get rid of my shyness and to confront people with my diabetes and even to provoke it.

The result is still amazing today. I never have to throw the subject of diabetes into the room or impose it on myself. The people around me always come to me out of their own interest and ask so many questions that make it easy for me to explain what type 1 diabetes is and requires.

Sharing my grape sugar supply with colleagues of mine is just a small and probably inconspicuous example of how diabetes strengthens my social skills. One is almost happy that I always have a "secret emergency supply" of sweets.

Everyone around us has seen us drink juice hectically or "choke down" dextrose in the case of severe, sudden hypoglycemia. But they have also seen us just as often jogging around the park with others, going to parties, taking part in long conferences, and pushing overtime without a break.

For all of us, we are sure that in case of an emergency, every one of our friends would know what's going on and whether they should ask, offer or insist sugar, or better call the emergency doctor. That gives each of us security.

This safety is the basis for us all to go through life without fear, despair, and self-pity.

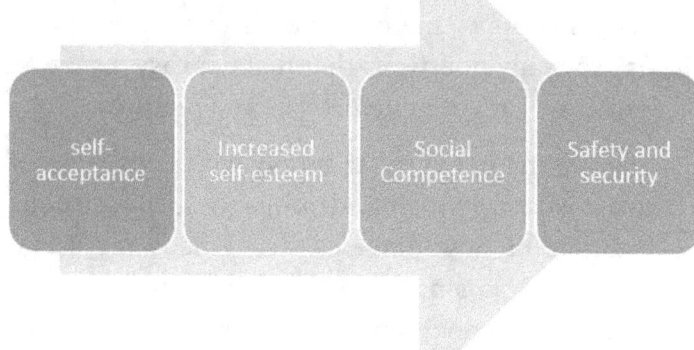

Having self-acceptance gives us the ability to speak with opinion and intelligence about how our condition is handled in everyday life. From this experience we have also been able to observe the above-mentioned pattern in other diabetics.

Think about each of these steps for yourself.

Start with the following questions:

- Do you fully accept your "diabetes fate"?
- If not, do you wonder why?
- What would help you?
- What are you most afraid of or worried about?
- What countermeasures could they remove?

CHAPTER 4

THE IMPORTANCE OF HEALTHY BREAKS

It is by no means out of the question to allow oneself a time out, particularly frequently as a diabetic, "only" because one has a chronic illness. In contrast, the previous chapters focus heavily on strength and on the fact that one should consciously make oneself measurable with one's healthy fellow human beings. With my "relativity of truancy" I force this philosophy. I would like to emphasize how consciously and conscientiously one should deal with breaks in order to strengthen one's endurance.

Imagine you give everything every day and always work so hard that each day becomes increasingly more and more difficult. Stress begins to reflect in a high blood sugar. Your diabetes can then be less and less regulated. You inject extra insulin all day against it and are then are left with various nighttime hypoglycemias as the receipt of your exhausting day.

Waking to treat a low glucose multiple times throughout the night leads to only little sleep. Next you find yourself awake again early in the morning heading to your job, in which you act as a hamster, trying to run as fast and successfully as your well-rested colleagues. Under these circumstances you can never - or at least only with great difficulty - outgrow yourself and shine, which in the long run is demotivating and exhausting. Which above-average achievements do you hope to accomplish? How much praise do you sometimes receive for your daily average performance, that in turn, costs an above-average amount of energy?

Remember from the previous chapter:

If you confidently sell your strengths to your environment and present them well, some of your weaknesses may be forgiven.

So turn the hamster wheel around.

For example, give approximately two hours at full-throttle energy and maximum effort and then recover again for 15 to 30 minutes.

Such examples to recover and revitalize your mind include the following:

- Take one lap around the block
- Treat yourself to a small snack between meals
- Switch the computer monitor to stand-by
- Turn the notifications on your continuous glucose monitor system off or to silent for the time being
- Call your significant other, relative, or close

friend to catch up
- Enjoy a cup of coffee
- Sit down in a quiet area to unwind thoughts
- Put on headphones and listen to your 3-5 favorite songs
- Or retire to an empty conference room to take a nap or perform stretch exercises

Removing yourself completely from your work environment for a short amount of time is beneficial. This gives you creative power and enhances concentration. It is useful for everyone, even those without diabetes.

This method can stabilize your blood sugar dramatically and in the end - although very few in your environment may truly understand - only your productive performance and your positive charisma counts.

Do you believe that all people in the workplace put in the same work ethic and produce the same results in 8 hours just because they have they are clocked in for the same time period?

With the method of regular, short interruptions at work, you counteract the fact that your diabetes is tedious and you may possibly be absent for a longer period of time. You also strengthen your immune system and also protect yourself from catching other illnesses such as the flu.

Since we can theoretically "fail" for a short period at any time due to illness - which we don't want, because otherwise we could be free from the prejudices of society - we should consciously exercise mindfulness every day and make intelligent use of our energy.

This has nothing to do with working slower or worse, on the contrary. Let us not forget the burden our diabetes has on us every day. Therefore, consciously slowing down and doing something for yourself and your health is beneficial for yourself, your colleagues, and your employer. Even though you may not have the right to take special breaks during working hours, e.g. to measure blood sugar or inject insulin, we find it absolutely recommendable and justifiable to take prudent breaks as a health-impaired person.

In Vivi's opinion, this handling serves primarily as a "repair", which promotes long-term well-being, contributes to improved health, and serves as a more efficient resumption of work activities. Hardly any employer would have anything against it if you also maintain your ability to work in this way. After two hours (especially at the computer), everyone should take a break.

Ashley and Emily's experience

As we work full-time as registered nurses, breaks are undoubtedly necessary. Unfortunately, sometimes breaks are not possible with the demands of our heavy assignment, even while working night shift. This can make it extremely difficult to manage our blood sugars. Using a continuous glucose monitoring system and visualizing our blood sugars on our watch is one thing we do to make balancing our blood sugars at work a bit easier. This will be explained further throughout this chapter.

It is important to schedule a meeting with your manager to request and agree on accommodations regarding your diabetes in the workplace. e.g., a scheduled break. We do not recommend going a whole shift (12-13 hours) without stopping for a brief time to monitor your glucose and replenish the body. Believe us, it has happened more frequently than we would prefer and we have certainly learned through experience. We no longer allow our bodies to suffer- we will kindly and openly ask a coworker to cover our assignment for the brief time frame our body necessitates. We understand it would cause more harm to not speak up and then require further medical assistance.

Another piece to mention to your manager is the potential that your body requires 15 minutes of uninterrupted rest following a hypoglycemia until your blood sugar rises to a safe level. **It is imperative for your manager, leaders, and coworkers to understand that hypoglycemia may cause you to be mentally or physically unstable.** If unstable, you should not provide direct patient care for the time being. Having these standards in writing and with people of authority keeps yourself and your work environment safe.

Although neither of us have yet to resort to the accommodations made, they are available for times of need. The more common experience at work involves treating our bodies to quick-acting glucose when noticing our blood sugars trending downward, before we each a state where we cannot think clearly. A coworker may regularly find us gulping down a juice or eating a quick snack when completing tasks between patient rooms, but we have never risked a low blood sugar or a patient's status.

Dexcom: A continuous glucose monitor

We use the continuous glucose monitor system, Dexcom, to our advantage. In addition to wearing an insulin pump 24/7, we wear our Dexcom device - an adhesive patch and transmitter connecting to small sensor wire inserted under the skin - with pride. The reusable transmitter wirelessly sends a blood sugar reading to our cellular app, now continuously, (used to be every five minutes) and displays in a graph. It is helpful to visualize blood sugar trends and data to make adjustments and tighten our control.

Having our blood sugar readings and trends visible on our wrist while working is time-saving and can be life-saving. Through seeing our blood sugar and current direction we are able to minimize and even avoid some episodes of hypoglycemia. If we are extremely busy at work and fail to recognize that our body is in need of sugar, watches are a great tool to have as a back-up. As soon as we are notified of a low glucose alert (set at 100 mg/dl) and we check to see whether we are trending downward as compared to the previous reading, we are able to replenish our bodies with sugar quickly. Additionally, we receive a notification if our glucose level is falling rapidly; this signals us to either treat before our glucose falls below target or also keep it in mind while running the hospital halls at work.

Receiving alerts from our dexcom devices has been extremely helpful in these certain situations when busy especially because it could be a result from many factors affecting blood sugar: a decent sized meal before work, exercise that may affect us hours later, lack of sleep, and you simply do not have the time or thought to keep a close eye on your glucose trend. Remember, it is your responsibility and of utmost importance to maintain your own so you can fulfill your own duties for others at work.

THE SEVERELY HANDICAPPED PASS

IN THIS TOPIC, VIVI EXPLAINS HOW, IN GERMANY, IT IS POSSIBLE AND COMMON TO OBTAIN A SEVERELY DISABLED PERSON'S PASS. THIS PASS OFFERS ASSISTANCE AND OPPORTUNITIES TO THOSE WITH LIVING WITH A CHRONIC ILLNESS.

Vivi's experience:

After 15 number of years living with type one diabetes, I applied for and successfully obtained a severely disabled person's pass. If an individual's degree of disability is labeled as 50 or greater, like myself, he or she is granted five extra vacation days per year. I set aside my extra "vacation days" to use for regular doctor visits and for when I need to "recharge my battery" in order to function as well as the healthy environment around me.

The pass offers a tax-saving piece as well. In Germany, the degree of disability leads to a proportioned pay-back by taxes and is structured as follows:

Degree of disability	Annual lump sum in Euro (€)	Euro to U.S. Dollars ($)
25 and 30	310	~350
35 and 40	430	~480
45 and 50	570	~640
55 and 60	720	~800
65 and 70	890	~1,000
75 and 80	1.060	~1,180
85 and 90	1.230	~1,375
95 and 100	1.420	~1,600

Wondering if you are classified as severely disabled? It is worth taking a look at the Social Code (SGB) IX:

"People are handicapped if their physical function, mental ability or mental health is highly likely to deviate for more than six months from the circumstances typical of their age and their participation in life in society is therefore impaired. They are at risk of disability if the impairment is to be expected."

The determination of the degree is by no means only about the type of illness, disability, or about a diagnosis, but always about a functional deficit for a corresponding duration (longer than six months) and the effect on participation in life in society.

Parents can even apply for childcare costs as a supplement to rehabilitation during rehabilitation stays. Parents of children with disabilities can have the lump sum transferred to them. In return, they must receive child benefit or a child allowance for the child (§ 33b Abs. 5 EStG).

If you are a young adult diabetic, you should decide carefully if and when you want to tell your employer about your disability card. You may have more chances of advancement if you avoid discussion about it at the beginning. I will explain more about this in Chapter 6 (Diabetes Business Etiquette).

Ashley and Emily's experience:

This opportunity was something that we have never heard of nor thought about here in the United States. We would certainly put the extra allotted days to good use with both, the numerous scheduled and the unplanned, types of appointments that accumulate each year, fitting in visits to the lab multiple times per year, and to utilize after nights in which we get less than an hour of uninterrupted sleep due to unexpected highs, lows, insulin issues, device malfunctions, etc. Having this resource available would relieve the stress we experience over scheduling appointment days around work 4 to 12 months in advance. It also allows time to fix the unexpected issues rather than rushing right back into work before normalizing what is most important: your health.

We found that in Germany "disability" is viewed more from a medical perspective and is often equated with illness. We further researched the social security disability insurance offered in the United States: two disability benefits are available for those to apply.

The Social Security Disability Insurance, (SSDI) is funded through employer payroll contributions. Nine million employed adults currently receive this benefit, which only accounts for four of every ten people who apply, appeal, and are eventually approved. One-fifth of these recipients are living in poverty. The other benefit that disabled persons of the U.S. can apply for is Supplemental Security Income (SSI). It is designed to provide the basic needs for those classified as disabled and of the lowest socioeconomic class. Currently, less than 5 million working age people qualify for

SSI and receive about $525 per month. For many, it is their only source of income. SSDI payments average $1,140 per month. The OECD states the United States is placed 30th out of 34 countries in international rankings for disability insurance and benefits.

This link provides an additional sample of a German citizen applying for and explaining their experience with a disability card:

http://bt.offensivethinking.org/blog/2014/03/16/disability-passes-in-germany.ht

CHAPTER 5

PARTY ON! - DIABETES & PARTIES

ABOUT BASIC PROCUREMENT, DIPS, AND PEE-BREAKS"

If you suffer from type 1 diabetes as a child or adolescent, it is difficult to celebrate the first parties, disco, and bar visits with caution as you grow up and important to prepare them according to your condition.

Vivi's experiences:

I understand this very well, because I was only 21 years old when I was diagnosed. Diabetes could not limit my party mood at that time. I played down the disease and only slightly withdrew myself. From today's point of view, I took it all a little too lightly.

My little clutch had room for cigarettes and mobile phones, but no room for my diabetic supplies. "I can manage without all the stuff for a few hours," I told myself cheerfully (today I would say I was "frivolous" instead of "brave"). I was convinced that I could clearly feel hypoglycemia and counteract it with a fruity cocktail in time. During my party night I simply renounced carbohydrates in my eyes completely and accordingly I believed I did not need my insulin syringe.

I did not count the carbohydrates in the alcohol because I had always avoided cocktails and imagined that neither beer nor wine had a great effect on my sugar. My temporary feeling of freedom and just being like everyone else around me was a game with fire.

Alcohol, loud party music, and the many lights surrounding you quickly and imperceptibly cloud your senses, therefore your ability to recognize a low sugar may be blocked. If, for example, you became unsteady on the dance floor in a club or are speaking incomprehensibly, ignorant people would simply declare a diabetic with hypoglycemia drunk or stoned.

Ashley and Emily's experiences:

Being diagnosed at such a young age, we had a lengthy amount of time to gain knowledge from our endocrinologist before we reached the age of 21. Throughout this chapter we will stress the importance of responsibility and safety while drinking with diabetes. We are hopeful our experiences will provide you with useful insight for yourself, a loved one, or someone that is new to drinking alcoholic beverages with diabetes.

Our initial experiment with alcohol was much different than Vivi's. We both made certain that our Dexcom devices, our continuous glucose monitoring systems, were fully functioning. We wore our Dexcom devices all throughout college and still continue to wear them daily, especially if alcohol is in the picture.

Different types of alcohol affects each of us differently but the two most important facts are to keep an eye on your blood sugar and have all necessities along with you.

Diabetes is often overlooked because of ignorance and can potentially be fatal if proper first aid is not provided. If you are unlucky or not cautious, you may risk your life with the wrong "party behavior " as a diabetic.

In the following points we would like to clarify where the dangers hide and which tricks you can use to counteract these.

DIABETES & ALCOHOL

The unknown carbohydrate content and the amount of alcohol in the beverages are mainly responsible for the imminent danger of alcohol. While the carbohydrates cause the blood sugar concentration to rise rapidly, the alcohol has an opposite effect with a delay of about four to six hours. It takes almost an eternity to be noticed in the blood sugar.

In addition, the alcohol blocks the normal formation of new sugar in the liver. This means that alcohol consumption first causes the sugar to drop and then, after several hours, increase again irregularly.

If you drink more than one glass, it becomes calculatedly difficult to understand what mechanism one's metabolism goes through and when and how much sugar is channeled into the blood.

In addition, you don't necessarily sit on a bar stool during party nights (that's what you do when you get older ;)). Instead, you are constantly moving around, singing, and dancing, which in turn reduces an unknown amount of sugar.

In my (Vivi's) opinion, the biggest mistake in alcohol consumption is to attempt to calculate a fixed carbohydrate unit to administer the appropriate amount of insulin.

Both insulin AND the delayed effect of alcohol lower blood sugar and the diabetic will most likely run into a state of hypoglycemia. Then, if he/she consumes a sugary drink and absorbs it, after a few hours the sugar from the alcohol comes on top and you are back in a hyperglycemic state. Accordingly, the diabetic starts again with the counter-regulation ... and so on.

If the affected person is "out" during all these events and still celebrating, the party is everything besides relaxed for him/her. Furthermore, this sugar curve (up, down, up, down ...) simply doesn't end and comes with a lot of danger when you fall asleep intoxicated. Although we are not encouraging anyone to party often or excessively, following one's recommendations of completely renouncing alcohol or enjoying it with just one glass is simply unrealistic for young adults.

Vivi took the example of many conventional diets in which you can have a so-called "Cheat Day" per week. On this "Cheat Day" you can eat and drink anything you wish. This idea is under the premise that if you resume your diet on the following day, you do little harm to your diet success - if any at all. Everybody and every organism is different.

From this she has deduced that one wouldn't do much damage to their diabetes if well regulated throughout the week with appropriate blood sugar values and possibly accept one day of increased values - if a party is on the agenda.

Ashley and Emily can attest to those statements. If you are drinking cautiously and taking appropriate measures, your blood sugar may be no different than on a normal night. It is okay to celebrate periodically. You do not need to "hold back" from partying because of your diabetes; however, you may want to "opt-out" or be the designated driver for the night if your blood sugar values are uncontrollable that day/week. Use your own judgment, the help from your healthcare provider, and blood sugar trends to determine what is best for you. Alcohol affects everyone differently and you know your body best. Responsibility is key.

OUR MASTERY STRATEGIES FOR PARTIES:

Carry your diabetes supplies with you. If necessary, take them out of the "sugar bag" so that the individual parts can be stored more easily and slim in a handbag.

The minimum supplies in your bag/purse should include:

- Glucometer with lancet device and test strips
- Insulin syringe and 1-2 syringe heads/needles as spare, whether on injections or pump
- At least 2-3 packages of dextrose or quick-acting sugar
- Emergency glucagon kit

If you manage your diabetes with an insulin

pump, it is not a bad idea to carry either a syringe and insulin vial or extra adhesives and a pump set with you as a precaution. If you dance/move a lot and perspire, the patch may come off and cause the catheter to dislodge. This will prevent insulin from getting into your body and can lead to severely high blood sugar and ketoacidosis.

Start with a good foundation.

Do yourself a favor and eat some real food before the party. You will set yourself up best if the meal is well balanced with carbohydrates, fat, and protein. If the meal is made up primarily of carbohydrates, it may result in a BG spike followed by an inconsistent pattern throughout the night.

Drink a glass of water for each glass of alcohol.

Always drink a glass of water between your alcoholic drinks. On the one hand, it helps you to not dehydrate and stay sober longer. On the other hand, it supports your sugar. If your sugar increases in the meantime, the water will help you to regulate your electrolyte balance and relieve your kidneys, which are more and more burdened with the higher sugar.

Measure regularly.

Keep an eye on your diabetes unnoticed. For

example, you may want to check your blood sugar each time you visit the restroom. Nobody in your environment will notice this and you will always know where you stand.

We (Ashley and Emily) periodically peek at our blood sugar on our watch and most of the time it is unrecognizable by others. When a friend does recognize us glancing at our Dexcom to see our sugar trend, they are not shy to ask, "How are you? Do you need sugar?", and it is comforting having their support.

Correct carefully.

If you exceed 200 mg/dL during your party night and decide to give insulin, you should correct carefully. Keep in mind: you are under the influence of alcohol.

I (Vivi) always handle it as if 150 mg/dL is my target and anything above that I correct. If I tend to sit around at a party and have a good time, I correct with my normal correction/sensitivity factor. If I dance a lot, I only take half the insulin dose because I probably break down the "remaining sugar" - as in sports - by exercising alone.

For us (Ashley and Emily), we typically do not cover for a high glucose while out at a party or bar. In addition to our high energy personalities,

ESPECIALLY when out celebrating with our good friends, we are aware of the delayed effect that insulin has on our bodies. From experience, we know that the partial doses taken for food/sugary drinks are enough when combined with dancing and the after effect that alcohol has on the blood sugar. Time and time again our nights have ended with a low blood sugar before bed or during the night. Our recurring experiences led us to change our technique and we now see fewer hypoglycemias post-party. It is better to see the rise and gradual fall of glucose trends than to immediately correct and chase your tail later. Everyone is different, so the same technique may not be the best for you. Staying aware and dosing cautiously when you drink is important.

Observe & individually optimize.

At the first few parties you attend, keep a close eye on your diabetes, alcohol, and snack consumption. On the following day, evaluate how you managed with your insulin administration. In this way you can develop your individual coping strategy.

Respect the support.

With our parents helping care for us since day 1 of diagnosis, they were a bit fearful to let go when it came time to leave for college. We respect our parents wish to support our diabetes management and "follow" our blood sugar trends on the Dexcom Share App. This app allows select people to receive notifications when one's blood sugar is out of range. It can sometimes it can be annoying to take the extra step and reassure them that we are okay and are taking the proper measures, but it can also be life-saving. It has been helpful to receive the extra alert through a telephone call during the night to wake up and treat a low BG. The lack of sleep from nursing school, sports and activities, and social life sometimes got the best of us and we have slept through alarms. We have gained responsibility through these experiences and have taken extra measures to overcome this challenge: placing a bluetooth speaker on the nightstand, sharing our glucose patterns with our roommates (each other!), laying our phones on a hard surface to intensify the vibration, and triple checking that our alarms are not silenced and phone ringer is on loud before falling asleep. It is a work in progress and we will always have goals to improve our diabetes management; this is one of them.

On the discussion of our mother "following" our blood sugars through Dexcom's share app, it sometimes caused her to worry during our college years when she knew we were out drinking and she received a low blood sugar alert. There have been multiple occurrences in which we had to exit the party scene to find a quiet place to call her and let her know we were okay. Sometimes we felt that is was an unnecessary, extra step, but we realized it beneficial for all of us. It helped us to keep an eye on our glucose trend and also helped our mother out by easing her worry when we showed that we were on top of it and being the responsible adults that we were.

In other words:

How do our tips work for you??

- Can you keep your sugar stable?
- Are you quick on correcting over 200 mg?
- How do the modified corrections work?
- With what blood sugar do you fall asleep and wake up?

After some "celebration practice" you will have your own specific blood sugar targets and know how much insulin you need to enjoy your parties with confidence.

DIABETES & DRUGS

ENDANGERMENTS & CONSUMPTION FEELINGS

I, Vivi, have tried only cannabis several times in my life. In a training with other diabetics I learned more about the use of cannabis and experience with other drugs.

The following characteristics could be observed by type one diabetics when using drugs:

- Fast pulse
- Increase in blood pressure
- Dizziness
- Pupil dilation
- Sickness
- Extreme thirst or appetite
- Sudden listlessness and limitless exhaustion.

Notice anything?

All the symptoms of intoxication associated with drug use are also found in diabetology.

The sugar slipped into my cells after a joint at a dangerous 28 mg/dl. Everyone around me was stoned and nobody reacted when I heard the alarm shortly before the loss of control. By my own efforts I quickly gulped a lemonade and saved myself from hypoglycemic emergency.

The confusing thing for me was that I had used cannabis before without any side effects. So why did I feel so bad that one time?

Let me remind you that drugs do not comply with pharmaceutical guidelines. They are always mixed differently- depending on where you get them from. They may be mixed more and sometimes less strong or pure. The effect on one's own body and thus on diabetes is correspondingly unpredictable.

Even more important than alcohol consumption is awareness in dealing with drugs. I do not want to write here how or what you have to prepare when you use drugs.

But just remember to have everything you need in every situation- especially for sudden hypoglycemia. Even experienced diabetics find it almost impossible to react in time to maintain control.

CHAPTER 6
DIABETIC BUSINESS ETIQUETTE

APPLICATIONS

If you google the topic "Diabetes and job applications" or "Diabetes in job interviews" you will be immediately informed that you do not have to mention your diabetes. Basically, it is recommended to you directly and without digression not to say a word about it and even better not to mention it.

Many employers have little or no experience in handling this illness and it may cause uneasiness and fear. Some employers still consider diabetics to be less efficient and risk-prone today - and may therefore send you a rejection if they know about your illness before getting to know you personally. Nowadays, employers include non-discrimination acts posted in the job description and application that should provide reassurance that your diabetes will not lessen your opportunity.

One thing is for sure:

The concealment of his diabetes in the interview is not a reason for dismissal!

According to the jurisprudence of the German Federal Labour Court (BAG), a "health question" of a general nature without a concrete reason is not negligent.

But beware, there are exceptions here as well: *Questions about the applicant's state of health are permissible if the illness "either significantly impairs or nullifies" the applicant's suitability (BAG, 2 AZR 279/83).*

Such questions are thus permitted in exceptional cases, i.e. if they would lead to an immediate, concrete danger for the applicant or for third parties when carrying out the activity. This includes certain professional groups, such as commercial pilots or police officers with firearms. In this context, it is important to know that it is punishable to withhold information from our diabetics if we already know at the time of application that this job is out of the question for us due to illness.

But back to the normal case:

I, Vivi, recommend an application and an interview without mentioning your diabetes. Your illness says nothing about your ability and suitability to do the job you are looking for. In an interview, it's all about pricing yourself into the company you're looking for - selling yourself.

Now think of supermarkets .... Goods with an expiration date or damage will be sold or sorted out cheaper. So why should you give yourself such a stamp if your abilities are at least as good as those of your competitors?

I even go one step further. You are different from your competitors. Emphasize it and make yourself stand out instead of being submerged in the crowd! While damaged goods are sorted out or put on a "junk heap", "individual items" are sold at higher prices and displayed as something special in showcases. Which "object" would you like to embody?

From another aspect, mentioning your condition could be beneficial to include in "interview talk" if it is relatable to the position you are applying for (for example, a job in healthcare). If using your experiences with diabetes to mention strengths, we recommend to be open about it. Also if diabetes influenced your decision to pursue a certain career, be sure to mention that if it is important to you!

In fact, those with type one or even a relative of type one may have some positive experience that can separate you from others. Use your management and organization skills, dedication to yourself and keeping others healthy, and your motivation to never give up to your advantage...you work hard for it!!

The design of your written application:

This following section was written by Vivi to provide recommendations that may be useful when starting the application and interview process of a career.

Recruiters primarily pay attention - within seconds - to the following things:

- Does the application have all the required content (resume, certificates)?
- Are the key qualifications immediately recognizable and compatible?
- Does the application have a uniform and well-structured format?

<u>It is recommended to create everything in one PDF document:</u>

Cover page

- Include name, contact details, & date of birth
- If necessary, add a motto or a guiding principle to your cover page under which you are active or which gives a meaningful description of how you work.
- Example: "Teamwork makes the dream work!"

Overview / summary of your key qualifications

- A maximum of 3 to 5 points, which you most likely have in common with the job advertised.

  TIP: Have a look at the structure at www.LinkedIn.com. Here, too, people like to work with "tags" to make it easier for recruiters to find suitable employees and managers.

Resume

- Include most recent activities first!
- Always specify the months and years with experience and employment periods.
- Emphasize what needs to stand out, i.e., put company and position in bold and possibly a larger font size.

Testimonials: ONLY THE MOST IMPORTANT TESTIMONIES!

- **Layout:**

  Do you have little work experience? Consider portrait format and font size 12.

  Do you have a lot of work experience? Landscape format, in column form and font size 10.

This will save you space and you will not get a thick "application catalogue", but a slim, handy and above all clear application folder.

Tips:

- Take a close look at the job description and select the keywords so that you can include them in your advertising later.

- Find out about the company, philosophies, and perspectives on the company homepage.

- What do you particularly like? What makes the company different?

- You can integrate such things intelligently into your cover letter later.

- Make sure that you "know" your contact person! The Internet and the business platforms mentioned, such as XING and LinkedIN, allow you to get to know the companies and contacts better in advance. Browse through their pages and websites to find out about their private and professional interests and backgrounds.

After all, it has never been wrong to speak the language of those who want to be heard!

OUR TOP TIPS OF A SUCCESSFUL DIABETIC APPLICATION/INTERVIEW:

1. Sum up your strengths in your written application. Create profiles on business portals such as XING and LinkedIn that are compatible with your company and job you desire. These platforms give you a "360°" profile as an applicant.

2. Keep your illness to yourself during an interview and concentrate instead on your abilities, strengths, and competencies. NO questions about health impairments.

3. If you are not sure whether you are allowed to work in a particular profession with diabetes, consult your endocrinologist or do your research beforehand.

4. Prepare yourself particularly well for the company and the interviewer- professionally as well as privately.

5. Be your own salesman. Think in advance which of your qualities and abilities are most important to the company so that you can highlight them in the conversation. Furthermore, you should bring along a brief list of prepared questions that YOU would like to ask the company! It is quite exciting if you dare to ask challenging questions - for example asking about negative Internet valuations, falling share prices, high fluctuation, or competitors.

6. Turn off your mobile phone respectfully! At the beginning of your interview, place a folder, a printout of your application, the job advertisement, as well as a pen on the table!

7. Don't forget to always smile with confidence, say "please & thank you", greet and say farewell with a firm hand, sit straight and upright, and always keep eye contact!

8. Prepare yourself with plenty of time beforehand to stabilize your blood sugar in attempt to avoid a severe high or low blood sugar throughout the interview.

9. Measure your sugar unnoticed BEFORE the interview (e.g. in the bathroom). Assume that the interview can last at least 60 minutes. Avoid hypoglycemia and keep your sugar a little higher (e.g. at 150 mg/dL) to have a "buffer" if it may decline.

10. If you ever feel sick or become dizzy in a conversation (happened to me before), then smile friendly and say something like: "Now I was apparently a bit excited in advance. Could I have a moment before we continue?"

11. If you have an apple watch/smart watch and are wearing it as an accessory (remember your phone should be off), make certain it is set to "do not disturb". You will survive without your CGM readings during the interview!!

CONFERENCES & PRESENTATIONS

From your education, studies, or professional experience, you may already know much about practical conferences and presentations - as a participant, host, or initiator. Before I (Vivi) became a diabetic, I was someone you would generally call an "attention magnet". I was not upset by anything, had an answer to everything, and was never at a loss for a quick saying that made everyone laugh or pause. After my illness, I was initially insecure and no longer able to explain my charisma, affect, and ability to communicate. I thought about how to be the center of attention without being "actually seen by myself".

So if I was a competent but rather impulsive speaker before my illness, it was clear to me that I would have to prepare myself better with my diabetes. It was my plan to deceive beyond uncertainties and to be perceived and appreciated with the same professionalism. Under no circumstances did I want to pay attention to possible weaknesses or even be reduced to them because, in my opinion, it would hinder my career.

Now you may be wondering what insecurities I'm talking about. Let me give you an insight into the diabetic emotional world:

At conferences or presentations as a host/moderator or simple speaker, you have stage fright, sweaty hands, thirst, a racing pulse, etc.

- These are all symptoms that we also feel with a drop in blood sugar, which can upset you if you don't have the ability or time to measure your glucose.
- You may have a presentation/conference lasting more than 2 - 3 hours in length, during which you cannot leave a room and may stand in front of an audience and are being observed by others.
- It can happen that the thought only revolves around your blood sugar and you lose your concentration and the thread.

Food and refreshments are served often at meetings and conferences - perhaps before or after the event. There may be only unfavourable drinks, e.g. only juice and cola instead of water. I (Vivi) have also experienced pizzas or sandwiches being delivered to the conference room due to a lack of time for a real break.

- Diabetics should eat regularly. But if you want to avoid injecting insulin, you have to avoid carbohydrates. This, in turn, can lead to loud stomach rumbling or hypoglycemia after several hours.

- If you are the center of attention, you are often held up and addressed during breaks or followed by colleagues to the bathroom.

You may find it difficult to retreat to measure/treat the sugar unnoticed. Receiving questions and astonishment about diabetes can perhaps accumulate more rumors than the actually accomplished achievement. This can lead to internal anger or even spoil your publicity/advancement. For this reason, I advise you to distinguish yourself through meticulous preparation. Play through all the possibilities in advance and prepare yourself accordingly!

- Where does the conference or presentation take place?

  In an office, event building, hotel?

- What does the program agenda look like? What breaks are planned?

- Is the list of drinks or meals known? Who could you ask? (Many people provide it today because of allergies)

- Ask about the type of execution or plan for the meeting/conference.

- If necessary, always take your own water or fruit and quick sugar with you.

- Are there several bathrooms there - perhaps

on different floors?

- If there is the possibility of several floors, plan in advance your walk to another area or bathroom than the mass.

- What alternative possibilities do you have if you don't find a retreat?

    Example: Staging an urgent cell phone call for which you need the building or room.

Overall, we recommend that you start a longer conference or presentation with a slightly increased sugar level (approx. 150 mg) if possible. Due to the excitement during your presentation, it is quite possible that you will also burn more and reach your target value of 100 mg after 1-3 hours. With 150 mg you do not have a real risk value, but you do have a buffer that makes you appear self-confident because you should be protected from hypoglycemia for a longer period of time.

Furthermore, I (Vivi) will provide you with the following organizational and content-related tips, which will give you a perfect basis for preparing successful conferences and presentations. If you are prepared for all eventualities, you are guaranteed to step up just as spontaneously, impulsively and confidently as before your illness!

GOLDEN RULES

Organizational:

- If possible, place a bottle of water and - depending on the length of the lecture - perhaps a juice (for emergencies) on the speaker's desk before the start of the event.
- Introduce yourself before you start talking.
- Then welcome the participants with a round of introductions.
- Present your topic and briefly explain the organizational aspects as a moderator.
- Make sure you don't see confidential or private content when you share your entire desktop - especially about your diabetes.
- Arrange in advance (also with the organizer) how much time can be taken for questions or discussions in the aftermath of your presentation. This will tell you how long you need to keep your sugar stable without food. If necessary, prepare an alternative where participants can continue their questions and discussions with you outside the conference. (e.g. chat or break room at a designated time).
- A perfect conference ends with the follow-up and a meeting report or minutes.

Verbal:

- Make sure you have a positive basic attitude: keep going through your presentation in your mind and visualize that everything will run smoothly and successfully.

- Practice your lecture on timing, voice modulation, pauses, meaningfulness & understanding as well as humour - best with a rehearsal lecture in front of friends.

- Observe the law of a good first impression: How do you earn sympathy points? E.g. in the introduction round.

- Present credibly and with commitment. Maintain eye contact with the audience and try to make everyone feel that they are important.

- Practice open gestures, friendly facial expressions, a calm look - the better you are prepared, the less you (and your sugar) will be upset.

- Plan a certain dramaturgy into your lecture: Change your location in a targeted way and use your whole body to create excitement and the attention belongs to you.

- Speak vividly and effectively. Be careful to present slowly, clearly, with pauses in effect at the appropriate times.
- Keep the auditorium's attention at a high level, for example with anecdotes, cartoons, questions, or discussions that you have prepared and rehearsed beforehand.
- Avoid overloaded slides, unclear writing, slide changing too fast, and long sentences.

Last but not least:

Avoid personal questions with direct counter-questions or "move" it to "the next time". After your presentation, it is best to leave the word with the others. People love attention & recognition. Utilize this and you will be popular - and your diabetes is invisible!

CHAPTER 7

EXPERIENCE WANDERLUST

In this chapter, Vivi explains the basic ideas and her experiences of traveling abroad with diabetes.

Studying abroad, working abroad, or simply traveling around means first and foremost entering a new culture. You are open to it and are open to other customs and know that you will also find your way around a foreign language. Language, morality, history, law, economy, science, tradition, validity, action, and handling differ significantly from culture to culture. These are decisive things that - depending on your own adaptability and openness to learn - can influence your life abroad.

The previously mentioned cultural concepts affect every traveler abroad. But as a diabetic, of course, there is also our condition, which is more or less known in every country of the world and is treated completely different in many continents of the world.

In the Seychelles Islands, for example, it was claimed that there were no native diabetics. For this reason I would not have been able to obtain any medical aids or medicine on the spot without having learned this beforehand. By the way, I was six months pregnant at this time.

Therefore, no country in the world is an exclusion criterion for us diabetics. Apart from the cultural differences, there are only other precautionary measures to take, which will make your time abroad a bit easier.

After my studies, I worked for four years in the foreign service of the second largest tour operator in Germany. I was to be available around the clock for my job to support the travelers in all (possible and impossible) situations - even after death. I worked where others go on vacation. As dreamlike as this sounds, it meant being available 24 hours a day, 7 days a week, walking around in uniform and tight pumps in 40°C (104°F) heat, and driving broken cars without air conditioning, which could stop anywhere and at any time (e.g. in the middle of the stone desert of Egypt).

Like almost anyone who has spent a long time abroad, I can only confirm that it was sometimes the most valuable experience of my life - from nightmare to fantastic adventures like "1001 Nights", everything was there.

In the end, it is a time that I never want to miss but rather want to repeat at any time. My years abroad have taken me further, broadened my horizons, and made me more independent. The time abroad has helped me look beyond my own nose, build on my social skills, stand up for myself, organize myself and others, and not panic so quickly if something does not go according to plan. THIS all applies equally to the traveler as well as to those at home!

There are many things you can prepare before a stay abroad, but how it will actually work out on site, you will never really know 100% in advance. Let yourself be consciously involved and try to find solutions for your individual concerns on site with the help of flexibility, patience, talent for improvisation, and a good connection to your fellow human beings. For example, you do not always have guaranteed breaks abroad. Depending on the country and activity, there may be no breaks at all, only very short ones, or very irregular ones.

In addition, not every employer lets you decide where you should be deployed and sent, live, and work. The more openly you show yourself and give, the more conducive your career will be.

I have found that exotic target areas - which of course have greater respect and require a longer settling-in period - will later bring you more recognition. This is because not everyone dares to do it and of course it requires more pioneering work.

Speaking of exotic destinations...

Please never think that you can go anywhere, feel comfortable, know your way around, have people around you, and get started with your "integration program". In most cases, you need about two months to feel at home and to acclimate. Just reckon with it in advance and take your time.

In Turkey and also Egypt I lived in areas which looked like sand mountains without street names. I had to memorize how I came home and unfortunately in the beginning that often went wrong. Considering that, I worked sometimes more than 16 hours at a time and not only during the day. It was twice as hard to find my way home with extreme exhaustion and the changing daylight. Often the tears then came to me - which everyone likely has to overcome once.

If you come from Germany, you are used to a strong democracy, equality, and respect in every situation. Basically, you don't know that you are rejected or even ignored in negotiations. You may be shocked when people yell at you for trifles and trifles. Please take it calmly and always attempt to remain calm and polite. Building relationships is the key to success abroad and is time-consuming.

You may think it is not your way of doing business; however you do not want to change or humiliate yourself. If possible, discard these thoughts and feelings. It is by no means a devaluation of you as a person. It is only intercultural differences that you have to adjust to.

The same unfortunately applies to our diabetes. In Germany, people affected by diabetes are treated as normal as possible. In foreign countries, people are often not so well-informed and that is why some people try to educate themselves and keep control.

DECISION MAKING

Are you interested in traveling abroad for a longer period of time but aren't quite sure whether this is something for you? Then ask yourself the following questions:

- Why do I want to go abroad?
- How do I envision my stay abroad?
- Destination?
- Accomodation?
- Meals?
- Diabetes?
- Job?
- Freetime?
- Time of duration?
- Funding?
- Which country interests me most and why?
- What qualifications do I bring with me for my stay?
- Competences & Special Skills?
- What would I like to do abroad?
- Who supports me abroad or from my home country and how?
- What do I need to feel comfortable in another

country/place?

- How do I imagine the time after my return?
- What are the risks involved in my project?
- What does my health insurance cover? Can I take sufficient medicine with me beforehand for my stay or is someone from my circle of acquaintances/relatives authorized to procure and send me the medication as it needs refilled?
- What opportunities does this experience offer me?

Create a PRO & CON list and draw up a financial and task plan for your planned stay abroad. The financial plan should be as comprehensive as possible and cover the entire duration so that you can see how much money you will actually need in total. That is, similar to a "forecast", you write down all estimated monthly expenses in the foreign country as well as the expenses you have to make before you leave.

Think of as much as you can:

- Insurances & Rents,
- Current subscriptions and your cancellation periods,
- Clothing and shoes,

- Suitcase and backpack,
- Medicine, emergency equipment & cool box,
- Cell phones, cameras, computers, books,
- International Driving License,
- Learning and Preparation Courses

The task plan goes hand in hand with your financial plan and should also be carefully considered.

Then I advise someone to go over your list, put it through its paces, and go through it with you. This could be someone from your circle of acquaintances who has already gained experience abroad, for example, your boss or professional agents who organize and accompany such stays abroad.

I am also happy to help you with my voluntary mentoring programme via Skype, email, or phone.

"HEALTH"

The topic "health" should sometimes be the most important part of your planning. Plan early on to have your doctor examine you again properly.

Also find out whether any vaccinations are necessary for your destination.

I also recommend that you discuss a few individual arrangements with your doctor. These can look like the following:

- Can relatives/acquaintances accept and redeem information for the duration of your stay abroad?

- Is it possible to receive and redeem the prescription abroad at today's "online pharmacies & companies"?

- Is it possible to take all prescription medicines with you for the entire stay abroad in advance? (Such special regulations are possible with health insurance up to one year, but must be requested separately and supported by the doctor treated).

- Ask for a multilingual doctor's letter that allows and justifies you to take your medication with you when you travel (in some exotic countries you may otherwise be suspected of drug trafficking and smuggling).

- Inquire about support and exchange with your doctor via email, SMS, Messenger, or Whatsapp. There are situations in which you may want to question treatment methods abroad or your own well-being and need guidance.

- For information: Doctors are authorized to obtain extra costs (flat service rates) for care via email and/or mobile phone. However, not all doctors do this.

- In all cases, find out in advance about medical care in the country of your travel. Contact the Tourist Office or the Foreign Office for more information. Find out all the important telephone numbers and addresses in advance and carry them with you in your carry-on and luggage: emergency call, police, private or state hospital, pharmacies, your local and home contacts.

When I spent my first year abroad in Turkey, I was supposed to work in Marmaris, Dalaman region. But the airport there was still closed so I flew ignorantly to Antalya, where I only had a car and a map. For more than four hours, I drove through unknown and uninhabited landscapes with places I could not pronounce and people on the roadside with whom I could not communicate.

Something would have had to happen and I would have been completely lost. Today I would have been happy if I had a note with the most important telephone numbers and addresses that

I should have had at hand in case of an emergency.

CHECKLIST

So that you don't lose track of what you should do before your stay abroad, I have prepared a checklist for you. I hope this will make your planning easier:

Six months before departure:

- Check expiration of passport and apply for a new passport if necessary
- Apply for a visa.
- Register your residence or look for a new tenant.
- Cancel subscriptions & contracts (electricity & water, TV, telephone & Internet, newspapers/books, streaming services, mobile phone, etc.)
- Plan departure and outward journey - Now flight tickets etc. are still favorable.
- Find your vaccination card and receive any missing vaccinations.
- Talk to your endocrinologist now and, if necessary, start gathering your medicine.
- Clarify local medical care: Is the insulin you take available? Where and how can you obtain

it locally?
- Attend a language course.
- Obtain and engross yourself in travel guides.

Three months before departure:
- Apply for an International Driving License.
- If you are at a young age, organize International Student & Youth Card
    Foreign health insurance
    Accident insurance
    Liability Insurance
    Open a foreign account
- Look for accommodation abroad (best for the first month and then look for a permanent place to stay. This will usually be cheaper for you).
- Organize yourself a credit card.
- Check the validity of the EC card and check whether your bank has a cooperation center abroad.

One month before departure:
- Order cash in the local currency so that you

can at least bridge the first few days of your outward journey.

- Did you obtain a doctor's letter? Your diabetic ID card? How many drugs do you have together - how many months will that last?
- Select a blood group ID card or have it created.
- Ensure you have attended your routine visits: family doctor, dentist, podiatrist, ophthalmologist, etc.

One week before departure:

- Have a second key made for your home address
- Set up your mailbox/answering machine.
- forwarding request.
- Get welcoming gifts.
- Copy and translate the most important documents.
- Pack and weigh baggage - if necessary, register bulky baggage (less is more).
- Prepare who is taking you to the airport.
- Handover your apartment.

Experience and time has taught me that all countries - no matter where in the world - have good doctors and hospitals and that in an emergency you are treated as a German with a German health insurance card and insurance everywhere first-class. Furthermore, many things are easier if you don't think things through in advance but instead completely involve yourself in the new situation and the country.

Clarification is actually easier on the spot. Basically, you have to imagine your stay abroad as moving to another city of your same country. There, too, you have to build up a new network and this is often best done on the recommendation of other locals.

Don't be afraid and worry; instead, completely involve yourself in the new situation and firmly believe that there won't be any problems. There will be solutions, new experiences, and approaches you will gain.

Remember that as an employee or student you do not always have influence on your stay abroad or the destination. In most cases, the employer or the university will simply ask for your willingness and flexibility. The more open you are, the more career-promoting your stay abroad will usually be.

I probably wouldn't have wanted to move to Turkey, Egypt, or Tunisia back then. But once I had arrived, integrated and settled in, it made me feel like I was in exactly the right place. So let yourself be surprised and accept the challenge willingly!

If you are moving to a developing country, consider a few other details when planning and packing your suitcase:

We do not really think about hygiene like regular hand washing, because it is a matter of course for us and lack of water is an unknown phenomenon:

- Take disinfectant liquid with you (you can find it at the pharmacy for about one dollar per bottle) to keep your hands clean in case you don't have any water.

- Take wet wipes or damp washcloths with you, so that you can wash yourself with them if there is no running water available.

- Always have 1-2 liters of drinking water with you. You can cook with it if necessary or brush your teeth.

- Dry shampoo is a new trend. You can purchase it in drugstores, perfumeries, and hairdressers. It is also handy if you have a lack of water or just a certain amount of water that may not always be enough to wash your head.

- Think about how to keep your laundry clean and fresh without a washing machine. REI in a tube, gall soap, fresh spray (Febreeze) are good alternatives.

- At pharmacies we are used to getting everything or at least being able to order. As a rule, our pharmacies are even stocked within a few hours on the same day. Usually we are not familiar with the situation of not receiving medicine because it does not exist in the country.

- Inform yourself before departure about local pharmacies and their supply of medicine. Your doctor may be able to help you or give you tips. The Federal Foreign Office or tourist offices can also assist you. If, for example, your insulin is not available locally, you can discuss alternatives with your doctor in advance or even try them out.

- As a rule, you should trust the medical products in the visiting country and not take so much with you from your home country.

- When I lived in Egypt, many tourists fell ill again and again with the famous "gastrointestinal disease". I noticed that German products were worse or not working at all, while the local medicine was immediately effective.

- Nevertheless, I recommend that you take a

small "medicine chest" with you for longer stays. It should include:

    Pain tablets (for headaches)

    Throat pain pills

    Tape, bandage, disinfectant spray

    Bite Away (against mosquitos)

    Fennel & Chamomile Tea Bag

    Clinical thermometer

    Cold Pack

- Power failure is rare should this occur, the problem is quickly solved. Take matches and tea lights with you when you need them.

    Lighting sticks will help you to light up an entire room or even to draw attention to yourself if you are in need.

    You can buy fluorescent stickers. You can use them to stick on the most important drawers and find everything you need in the dark in the event of a power failure, such as your insulin or glucometer.

    Pack a flashlight with batteries or self-powered.

- Upon arrival at your destination, write down the number of your electricity provider or save it in your mobile phone. There you can ask when the electricity will work again. A mobile phone charger for your car can be useful to maintain contact with the outside world in an emergency.

- When you arrive at your destination, make sure you have a storage room with sufficient water and preserves, which you can supply for about one week in an emergency.

- Sometimes power outages are predictable. In such cases, fill the bathtub with water as a precaution. Then you can use it to flush the toilet.

- For us, nurses belong in the hospital. Just as much as nurses, fixed meals and a freshly made bed belong.

- It is not customary in every country to be entitled to a nurse. Even in Greece (EU) I experienced that relatives of the sick had to take care of the food and fresh bed linen.

- Find out about the treatment beforehand. If you can't think of anyone in Germany who could help you in an emergency and take care of you, talk to your health insurance company, your employer, or other contacts you have in the target area. If you do not have any contacts in the target area, try to contact someone online via a chat and discuss the issue.

- Theft happens everywhere. Your luggage can be lost anytime, anywhere. As a diabetic in particular, you should therefore have the most important things doubled and carried with you in your backpack.

- You should think carefully about your luggage distribution in advance and obtain a certificate from your doctor that you are allowed to carry your medicine in your hand luggage. In your backpack or hand baggage belonging (preferably sufficient for a bridging period of four weeks if necessary):

    Glucometer with an extra set of batteries

    Blood sugar testing strips

    Lancets

    Insulin

    Glucose tabs (min. 3 packs)

    Disinfection spray or gel

    Mobile

    Separate telephone and address book (you cannot always use your mobile phone abroad immediately)

    Laptop and / or IPad

    A clothing outfit for one day/night

    Toothbrush & toothpaste

Hairbrush & Moisturizing Cream

Money & half of your credit or debit cards (move the other half so you have something in case of theft).

Identity Card

Diabetic card in several languages

- The emergency call is always available in Germany and is answered with certainty within a few seconds.

- As we have seen in the example of the massacre in Tunisia in 2015, it is unfortunately not customary everywhere to answer an emergency call immediately and respond to it.

So think about who you can contact in an emergency.

Since I usually didn't know anyone in the destination area before my departure, I had this topic on my screen, but usually could decide on the spot in the first two months. An acquaintance I had then developed into a friend and I informed her about my diabetes. Furthermore, I always asked people if I could call them in an emergency and if they could help me.

Another advantage was that my friendships were locals who knew not only the language but also the system perfectly and could act and intervene accordingly.

With these examples I already imply the most serious differences which can exist in some countries compared to Germany and which should be experienced in advance.

The Federal Foreign Office or the tourist offices of the respective destination can always help you. In times of the internet it is also useful to research in advance or even to make friends before the journey and to ask locals how exactly what works.

ENJOY A HOLIDAY

The biggest difference to a longer stay abroad over a holiday is that you can take all the medicines you need with you. You can easily discuss and arrange this with your endocrinologist and the health insurance company in advance.

Furthermore, you don't need to worry about the medical infrastructure on site and you can prevent everything by riding ahead and equipping yourself with the necessary equipment. In addition to insulin, you should also consider vaccinations and foreign insurance.

In comparison to longer stays abroad, many people engage in above-average sporting activities during their holidays and indulge in intensive physical activities that would otherwise not be performed in everyday life.

Here are a few tips especially for your holiday:

1. **ADJUST INSULIN DOSE**

Remember in particular that your insulin requirement changes in the sun and especially during sport. Insulin can have a stronger effect on heat. The combination of sun and sport has an even more massive effect on your diabetic system, so that in the first few days you would rather inject less, observe your value, and correct it if necessary, instead of running the risk of severe hypoglycemia.

2. **DRINK A LOT**

Everyone loses more water when it's hot and when you're additionally active. As a diabetic, the increased drinking requirement is suitable for adding juice boxes, which also protect against hypoglycemia. Ashley and Emily want to include the importance of staying on top of fluid intake to decrease dehydration, which can contribute to ketoacidosis if ketones are present in the body.

3. **INSULIN PEN & PUMP**

With a lot of heat and perspiration, the cannula to the insulin pump occasionally stops working properly or ruins. Pack additional pump supplies and especially adhesives/tape. If you are not able to use tapes, diabetic athletes advise you to insert several pump sites in the morning to have the option to switch to a functioning one in an emergency. If you are on an insulin pump (such as the OmniPod) that you cannot insert more than one, be sure to carry extra supplies, insulin, and syringes with you.

If you are traveling with insulin pens, I recommend that you take a small, slim cooling bag for medicine with you before departure. The MedAngel temperature sensor is highly recommended. Ashley and Emily also suggest the Frio cooling bags for insulin. The cooling wallets are water-activated, come in different sizes, and affordable.

In all cases, we recommend that you take disposable syringes with you.

INSIDER TIP & ANECDOTE:

At the end of 2014 I flew to the Seychelles six months pregnant. The dream domicile welcomed us with 90% humidity. I managed myself with insulin pens for more than 12 years and only received an insulin pump since the beginning of my pregnancy from the recommendation of my doctor. My experiences in this respect were correspondingly low and so I took my old pen system with me in addition to the pump - "just as backup" I thought to myself. "Thank God", I say today!

The humidity in the air caused the body to perspire so strongly, even during light movements, that no adhesive in the world wanted to keep the cannula under my skin. After the 2nd day, I already calculated that the aids I brought with me would never be sufficient for the number of "catheter changes" that would be necessary. I had to insert a new catheter almost every 2-3 hours because of the situation, Panic ran through me - after all I was very pregnant.

I put on a fresh pump site for dinner in the evening - on as freshly as possible: showered, cool, and dry skin. It was perfectly supplied with insulin for dinner and overnight. In the morning I already saw the site adhesive was only half on me. For breakfast I pulled something tight over it - shirt or trousers - which pressed the pumps site against me, so that I could still deliver insulin by the pump for breakfast.

Basically, I let whatever happen after that... I left the pump site on until it released itself through the heat - only one hour after breakfast. From then I used my "old system" for the time being. I drank water constantly and kept active moderately but steadily with swimming, snorkeling, and taking long walks. Every hour I measured my blood sugar. With a glucose of 80-100 mg/dL, I ate a piece of fruit to keep me at a steady sugar level and at noon I ate low carbohydrate meal. If my sugar reached or went above 180 mg/dL, I carefully corrected through injection with my insulin pen and drank, as always, a decent amount of water.

It's hard to believe, but I had great blood sugar values and my pumping equipment lasted exactly until the end of my holiday vacation. I was so happy about it!

4. TIME DIFFERENCE

If you are traveling to a different time zone, discuss with your doctor whether and how you should adjust your insulin or tablet dose. If you're flying out west, the day will be longer, so you'll need more insulin. If you are flying to the east, the day will be shorter and you may need to lower the dose.

As we (Ashley and Emily) have traveled numerous times to areas of different time zones, it is essential to remember to change the clock time in your insulin pump. Our basal rate fluctuates every few hours, and if the time is not changed when switching time zones, it may result in extreme out of range blood sugars.

5. DOCUMENTATION

Although handwriting in a diary may not be for you, today there is also a lot of electronic support.

Data may be downloaded from your glucometer, insulin pump, or CGM device. Additionally, there are various applications on mobile phones that allow you to track your diabetes management. Sugarmate is one application we (Ashley and Emily) find useful. It continuously collects data from our Dexcom (CGM) account to provide additional information such as time and percent in range, Glucose Management Indicator (GMI) - estimated A1C level - and includes the option to input your own data such as carbohydrates and insulin. Reports can be generated through the app and delivered via email!

If you find it difficult to keep a regular list of your glucose levels, you should definitely try it on vacation. If something should happen, the doctors on site can help you better and provide immediate help.

Finally, I would like to give you the message that you should relax during your holiday - so don't let your diabetes get you down!

If something goes wrong, for example, if you lose your insulin abroad or spoil it, simply go see a doctor or find a hospital where you can get a qualified replacement. To be on the safe side, write down the trade name and the manufacturing company of your preferred product before you leave and note the symbol as

well as the production code of your product.
These designations are identical worldwide.

LONG TRIPS & FLIGHTS

Here is our approach:

- Always measure your blood sugar before starting your journey. This should be stable between 100 - 150 mg. If you are below 100 mg, eat a piece of fruit or drink a juice before the journey to be "on the safe side".

- Pack your car so that everything you need is reachable from the driver's seat.

- Juice may be best for emergencies (easy to open and quick to swallow. Dextrose is difficult to open with one hand at the wheel without being distracted - especially if you are trembling.

- Place your diabetes bag with all utensils on the passenger seat.

- Water and snacks should also be kept within easy reach - e.g. on the passenger seat or in the console.

- If you are flying, take dextrose tablets or fast-acting sugar such as skittles instead of juice due to the ban on taking liquids! You should also take a snack with you in a backpack or handbag and of course your diabetic test bag.

- When driving, plan regular breaks in which you can measure and eat your blood sugar in peace. Not only is it healthier, it also gives you more peace of mind.

- If there is an accident and then a legal question or legal dispute, a well-maintained blood sugar diary will help you.

- If you get sick on board while flying, never be ashamed to discreetly inform a stewardess. She can keep an eye on you or stand by you, help you to calm down, distract you, or give you something to snack on. I (Vivi) experienced this on a long-haul flight from Frankfurt to Bali. The more you have the feeling that something is wrong, but you can't correct it or locate it, the worse the feeling of helplessness and panic will get.

- Be aware that you are never alone on the plane. There is a high probability that there will always be a doctor or someone with medical expertise on board who can be located in an emergency. Furthermore, the stewardesses are professionally trained. In case of doubt, they can always talk to a specialist via radio.

- If you are driving alone for a lengthy period, keep someone aware of when and where you are going. It is always good for someone to know where you are if something should happen. Send a small "SMS" on departure and arrival and prearrange an action plan if this "SMS" does not arrive after some time.

- Do you have a speakerphone? Or can you connect your mobile phone with Bluetooth? Save the most important phone numbers under a speed dial. If you're not feeling well, make the quick call.

I had a similar situation on my way back from Dortmund to Frankfurt. At that time there were no mobile phones with navigation devices or GPS. My whole body was tingling with discomfort. I was still about 20 miles to the next rest stop and the snowstorm made it relatively impossible to hold it together. As I pondered about what I should say if I had to make an emergency call, I started to pay attention to where I was.

Always pay attention to motorway signs along your way, where you are, exactly where you are going, and how many kilometers/miles you are from different cities. Even if your mobile phone works, it can reassure you because it gives you back a bit of the feeling of "situation control".

TRAVELING WITH DIABETES: the short version

Aside from traveling abroad, here are the key points we keep in mind when traveling for vacations or short trips!

- Packing up your supplies

In addition to what you have handy and use frequently in your diabetic bag, be sure to have enough extra insulin, pump supplies, syringes, alcohol prep pads, glucometer batteries, chargers, adhesive swabs, tapes, lancet needles, testing strips, continuous glucose monitor sensors, and an extra transmitter. We have run into several instances when we didn't have one of these and had to problem solve. Try to always have an extra bag packed for travels!

- Refrigerator in your room?

Wherever you may be staying, call ahead and ask if there is a refrigerator in the room or if you can have a room with one. This is especially important for your extra (new vials of insulin) and warm places of travel such as the beach so your insulin does not spoil.

- Pharmacy nearby?

Always locate ahead of time where the closest pharmacy is. For example, I (Emily) once had ineffective insulin when on a trip to Colorado. This can cause panic and stress, especially if your "extra" insulin will not lower your BG. I contacted my doctor and she kindly ordered my normal prescription of insulin and also syringes to a nearby CVS. This worked out very well! A similar situation has happened when becoming ill on a trip. Emily was simply able to pick up antibiotics at the nearest pharmacy for an illness while in another state. Communication and having a good relationship with your doctors is so important!

- Family or close contact on standby

Again, make sure you make a couple reliable people aware that you are traveling. In addition to letting them know your travel itinerary, it is not a bad idea to share the hotel contact information. This way, they could contact the hotel if they have not received a response in a long time before investigating further. If there is an emergency, they will be able to locate the nearest hospital.

- Insulin in your bag

Just like we stressed the importance of keeping unopened insulin in the refrigerator, it is necessary to store the insulin kept with you in a cool place. The insulin may spoil, turn ineffective, or may not last as long. We use the "Frio" cooling bag which fit a vial of insulin perfectly. It is easily reusable and stays cool for days at a time. When on a beach or in very hot temperatures like while camping out, keep your insulin or pump in a cooler when not in use!

- Always carry extra low supplies!!

Low supplies (food with quick-acting sugar, low in protein and fat) to treat hypoglycemia should be with you or closeby wherever you go. This means in your purse (pocket for a male), in your car, in your CARRY ON luggage in addition to a checked bag when flying, and on your nightstand throughout the night. When staying in a hotel, I (Ashley) always have keep easily accessible sugar readily available on the table to grab during the night or to see and grab on my way out the door

- Is your wristlet/bag large enough to fit your necessary supplies?

Sometimes you may find this difficult, especially for sporting events, going out at night, or traveling and exploring when you don't want to carry any more than your phone and credit card; however this is so important! If you are just going out for an hour or two, take the necessities and keep the extra supplies accessible in the car or at the house/hotel if you are able to return when necessary. Essentials to us include your glucometer, insulin pump, testing strips, lancing device, 1-2 alcohol swabs, a syringe, and fast acting carbohydrates. You can always and usually easily find a soda or batteries if you run out!

If your BG tends to drop pretty quickly which could place you at risk to fall to an unconscious state, we suggest carrying the emergency glucagon kit with you at all times as well. You know your body best and if there is a chance you might need it or not. For us, we always carry it with us during the day if our bag allows it or if we may be spending the night out. Most of our purses fit the little red kit, but if not, we make sure to stay extra on-top of our blood sugars for the time being.

- Syringes!

As previously mentioned, having syringes are necessary in case a pump or insulin site malfunctions on shorter trips. If you are on pens or MDI, a disposable syringe is another form of your typical dosing and could be useful during malfunctions. This is also sometimes an easier and more compact way of carrying supplies with you rather than your pump supplies. Also, we occasionally take small dose injections with a syringe if our BG is running stubbornly high and not coming down. Sometimes it is not worth an entire pump site change but rather first trying an injection and evaluating if the problem resolves. You must be very careful with this technique, however, and understand your correction factor and "insulin on board". Always consult with your endocrinologist before trying for the first time.

CHAPTER 8
LIVING ALONE WITH DIABETES

The number of single-person households is increasing worldwide. In 2014, their share in Germany and Austria was already around 37%. The number of single-person households in the U.S. was recorded at 28% in 2013 and has also been on the gradually rise. The particular challenge for us diabetics is that this disease harbors risks such as hypoglycemia at night.

Especially for those who live alone, it is of fundamental importance to recognize the symptoms of hypoglycemia (tremors, dizziness, hunger, etc) promptly and clearly in order to prevent unconsciousness.

Although one may not be living alone, perhaps the individual works night shift like us (Ashley and Emily). When working night shift you must sleep during the day, which is usually when nobody else is around! These same steps apply to safely prepare ourselves and our surroundings.

It may bring fear and restrictions to live in these various situations for all who are ill and stand alone; however, just the opposite can happen! You can minimize your risk and increase your self-confidence and feeling of security if you consciously prepare for emergency situations.

Here are some coping strategies:

1. **Emergency Supplies**

In addition to your handbags and jackets, you should stock up on various things in your household for emergencies. The bedside drawer is suitable (perfect) for dextrose, the refrigerator for juice, and if necessary, the living room or pantry for gummy bears.

2. **Telephone numbers**

Store the most important phone numbers in your phone and place your phone on the bedside table when sleeping. Speed-dial numbers are also suitable for emergencies. Have these readily available for yourself; duplicating the contacts and phone numbers on a paper may be useful to have in the case that a first responder may need to contact someone.

3. **Third home emergency system**

Anyone can apply for a home emergency call system through the Red Cross. You receive either a "bracelet" with an emergency call button or a switch that you can place or mount anywhere. The advantage to this not needing to make any telephone call in an emergency. You press the button and an ambulance will be on its way to you immediately!

TIP: The Amazon device ALEXA can also dial stored numbers and the emergency call for you on command.

4. Diabetes Pass

Always carry an identity card with you that is easy for strangers to find in an emergency. If you are no longer able to inform someone before you lose consciousness, your badge can simplify and above all speed up first aid procedures!

Alternatively or additionally, you may choose to wear a fashionable medical identification bracelet, watch band, or chain. Some of the various Instagram accounts that manufacture chic, medical identification products include: @getmyid, @sofiancy, @Laurenshopeid, @myabetic, @poppymedical, @stampingstreet, @americanmedicalid, and @thoughtblossom.

5. Blood Sugar Log

It is helpful to record your glucose legibly on paper or electronically. In unsafe situations, we measure our blood sugars more frequently, i.e. every half hour to every 2 hours, or visualize it more frequently on the CGM. We (Ashley and Emily) at time screenshot our Dexcom CGM graph when we notice our sugars to be "all over the place".

I (Vivi) personally write everything on a sheet of paper. I also like to write down my feelings (dizziness, nausea, etc.) and note my insulin levels and anything that might be helpful for foreign helpers if I should no longer be able to communicate myself. I keep the piece of paper near me, depending on where I am at the moment!

6. Plan Activities & Equipment

When I do sports or go on excursions, such as a hiking day, I always make sure that my initial blood sugar level does not correspond exactly with my ideal target value but has some "buffer". At 150 mg/dl I feel stable to start an active day. Depending on the activity, I take sugar with me.

If you manage your diabetes with an insulin pump, we (Ashley and Emily) suggest decreasing your basal rate temporarily. Through trial and error with adjusting our basal rates, we discovered it is most efficient when decreasing it about half an hour prior to physical activity. The amount/percent to decrease depends on the intensity of activity, length of time, starting blood sugar, passed time since the previous intake of carbs/protein, and the amount of insulin still active in the body.

For longer or day-long activities, I (Vivi) keep a lot of liquid in my luggage, e.g. spritzers/juice. I add some sugar to my body at regular intervals and keep myself stable: approximately a juice box per hour. I always have dextrose, fruit, pure juice, muesli or power bars with me.

Nevertheless, I always try to take a look at my hiking routes in advance and estimate how long it will take me to get to the next alp and when and how many breaks will probably be necessary! The better prepared I am, the safer and better the day will go! Our thought: it is better to stay a bit higher when you're active!

7. Inform Contacts

When I travel or go on excursions I always tell some friends or acquaintances what I am doing. I ask them to call me at a certain time or on a certain day or to stop by to make sure that everything has gone well and that I am well.

8. Cultivate a trustworthy person

If you do not live in the immediate vicinity of your parents, you may know the feeling of insecurity if your mom or dad doesn't seem to be available for a longer period of time. How would you like to be able to get in touch with someone in your immediate environment and ask them to take a look at what's going on?

Such a trustworthy person is of gold-value for you, especially if you are single. Someone who just regularly says "hello" and looks after you. If you get into an emergency situation unnoticed, such a person can save your life. Talk about the topic just as openly and honestly and inform this confidant what to do in an emergency or who has to be contacted.

Are you prepared? Well then enjoy your single household without reservations!

DIABETES IN A RELATIONSHIP – AN OPEN WORD

When you get to know someone you have great interest in, you first and foremost want to show your best side in order to inspire that person. A chronic illness is rarely the most popular introductory topic with all its "depths". Maybe you mention your illness - consciously or unconsciously - or perhaps the person will notice themselves that you have diabetes in the beginning. In the rarest cases one would explain this illness "in detail" or negatively as an affected person, right?

Many play diabetes down in the beginning. To put it in general terms, I would think that we diabetics try to play down our disease as harmless in the beginning in order to avoid minimizing our attractiveness - and thus our chances. In general, it is certainly not attractive to fall into the "house" with "problems". I (Vivi) have done a lot of research on this subject on the internet and have read about it in forums. I summarized the collected statements as follows:

If there are pre-existing illnesses, which impair the common future life and/or reduce the quality of life, e.g. not to be able to give birth or have children, to have a shortened life time or a forthcoming handicap, then one should address it immediately. Immediately means before it comes to a firm relationship, because it requires not only understanding, but also the support of the partner.

Incomprehensibly, however, I have also found diabetes several times in the listings on the grounds that it is also a chronic disease that would have an immediate and lasting effect on the couple's relationship and future. Diabetes can reduce the quality of life and the partner has to be considerate in the long run.

I contradict this above statement personally. However, in order to distance myself from my subjective view as a person affected myself, I asked various people about this topic. The following recommendations were given:

- In the getting to know phase one does not have to mention diabetes proactively; rather, manage as usual. It is better to be discreet at the beginning and go to the bathroom if necessary (preferably also as a pump carrier).

- Should it become foreseeably more serious between you and your partner, show courage and raise the issue of diabetes.

"As you may have noticed, I often go to the bathroom before the meal... I think you should *know that I have type 1 diabetes and have to give myself insulin regularly".*

- Avoid explaining too many details in the beginning. Be brief and make it clear that you are coping well with this disease.
- Only take risks in the conversation if you are asked proactively.
- Avoid dramaturgy in your presentation. After all, anyone can learn how to deal with diabetes - not only for you, but also for your partner. Therefore, introduce your partner slowly to the topic.

Of course I (Vivi) also discussed this topic with my partner and asked him how he judged it today - more than nine years later - to be with a diabetic. Does he have a lot of responsibility? Do I reduce his quality of life or his plans for the future?

No, no, and no again.

Certainly there are difficult times and there are also situations where my boyfriend was annoyed by me and my illness. For example, I had to adjust some plans because of a sudden hypoglycemia or I had to go to the hospital because of hypoglycemia or the opposite: hyperglycemia with ketoacidosis. These are rare exceptions. Every time I was able to help myself. The support of my partner in these situations happens voluntarily and out of love for me. I can also say the other way around that there are situations that occasionally annoy me about my - healthy - boyfriend.

The topics and situations we diabetics face are relatively predictable depending on how we handle our disease - while things happen arbitrarily in our hearts. Nevertheless, mutual support is the basis of a normal and healthy relationship. Accordingly, it is not possible to speak of an impairment of the quality of life or of the future for either one or the other. It is clear, however, that a partnership bears most fruit when no one feels "hoodwinked" or lied to. With this I would like to encourage you to speak openly. Stay true to yourself and if you embody your diabetes as part of your great self. There is objectively no reason to find you less attractive and great - on the contrary!

The same situation exists for Ashley and her significant other. Meeting in college, a lot went on between classes, cheerleading, studying, and our social lives! She did not hide checking her blood sugar, taking insulin, and all else that is done to manage diabetes. Thankfully her partner was open from the beginning to learn and was accepting of the fact that diabetes was just another part of our lives.

Bottom line: you should never be with someone that will not accept you for who you are. On the other hand, it is also important to appreciate all that your partner does and cares for you regarding diabetes. Type one diabetes has its challenges which may temporarily affect both the diabetic and the diabetic partner's plans. If not handled in the appropriate way, these challenges could take a toll on the relationship. We think it is best to keep your partner well informed and up-to-date on how you manage your diabetes but not bore or overwhelm them with too much information.

The key to this situation is explaining it at the learner's speed. There is so much to learn and teach about living with diabetes, you can't possibly tell them in a week! After almost five years, there are still new situations that arise frequently and which Ashley which explains to her boyfriend. Besides the basic and emergency situations, the best is a teach-as-you experience. Just like for your coworkers and acquaintances, you don't want to overwhelm, overexaggerate, or scare them! These individuals are the ones that will learn to understand you best, be there for the most difficult times, and stand by you through it all.

There have been occurrences where we have been caught with a surprisingly low glucose somewhere and do not have enough sugar on hand - on a run, out running quick errands, at a bar - and in an instant our significant others are on a mission to find the nearest sugar. A quick example: Ashley was enjoying her night out with her boyfriend and friends and received a sudden falling trend glucose alert on her CGM. She went up to a bartender to ask for a sugar-loaded soda and drank it quickly. Fifteen minutes later her blood sugar was still low. She turned around and saw her boyfriend at the bar already requesting a soda. How sweet!

When your significant other really gets to know you, they may start to realize when your glucose is high or low depending on your symptoms. For example, sometimes before we even think of it, our boyfriends have said "what's your sugar level?" and "you may want to check your CGM" when our actions mimics an out of range sugar - constant thirst, urinating frequently, speaking incomprehensibly, appearing pale, etc.

CONFLICTS & HOUSEHOLD CHECK

Regarding a healthy and balanced diet that you as a diabetic or as a reference person of a diabetic should pay attention to, there are hundreds of advice books available.

If you frequently have hypoglycemia and consume carbohydrates accordingly, a regular intake of healthy carbohydrates is indispensable to prevent this situation. I (Vivi) know this inner conflict very well. Although I am of normal weight, I have always wanted to be in "ultimate form" like the ladies on the high-gloss magazines. It's one thing to balance your diet. To reduce your caloric intake as a diabetic in order to lose weight, without falling into hypoglycemia, is a balancing act and not always easy.

Frequently I (Vivi) have faced hypoglycemia as a result of restricting carbs in the evening or at night. The carbohydrates that I then stuffed into myself broke my diet every time which very often made me angry. What annoyed me most of all was how I poorly controlled my carbohydrate intake in the intoxication of hypoglycemia.

With hypoglycemia, I often enter a state in which I feel as if I have no control. Can you relate?? The diet is forgotten, the healthy diet is forgotten... forgotten is the rule of thumb of how much carbohydrates one should actually consume in the case of hypoglycemia. It is basically "hands on food and in the mouth" until a pleasant, safe feeling appears. The certainty of having survived the hypoglycemia! This is then followed by a terrible feeling, because one can think all at once again clearly and notices the amount consumed in the last 10 minutes could equal as much energy the body needs throughout the whole day...

How one "diets" best and thereby avoids hypoglycemia will be explained in a later chapter explicitly. What will be discussed now is what you should have in your house or on hand if you suddenly fall into a state of hypoglycemia. We will tell you which portions you can take into account in advance so that you don't go from a low to high blood sugar, but directly to the target level.

It is important for your household check that you ALWAYS have a few things for emergencies at home if a sudden hypoglycemia overwhelms you or your relative. In this context, it is important to clarify the presence of certain basic foods with your "roommates"/family members.

Of course, anyone is welcome to the juice and bananas, but it must be clear that there is always something left for the diabetic - enough readily available to treat 1-2 hypoglycemias for each diabetic! As a diabetic, you have to clarify how this works and what quantities are involved.

Growing up, we (Ashley and Emily) classified certain foods in the pantry as diabetic-specific. Food items such as skittles, starbursts, clementines, and juice were placed in a specific location in which we all could locate in an emergency. We took on the responsibility (once around school-age level) of keeping these items stocked and making sure others were aware which snacks and sugar items were to be left in the pantry for us.

In addition, I (Vivi) want to provide you with my experience:

At first it was often difficult for my partner to leave anything. During a difficult time of blood sugars, before I went to bed, I always checked to see if my "antidotes" were still available in case of an emergency. I became "wild" when I noticed that there was nothing left. I sent my friend to the gas station to buy a juice or something similar for emergencies. I repeated the urgency of the supplies over and over again, until one day I really had a hard time with a low blood sugar without having something at home. My friend could not resist and had consumed my supplies. That was the moment when I dissolved household sugar in hot water to help me out and it was also the moment when my friend finally understood why I insisted that he had to leave me some food!

Low sugar for oneself feels weird. Some notice it because they feel dizzy, sweaty or shaky. Others have an absolute craving for food, which is especially dangerous because you tend to eat the wrong thing in excess. I belong to the last sort. Nevertheless, I try to "reward" myself in lower sugar phases - the lower sugar itself is already "punishment" enough. However, I always have a few things in my household so that regulation takes place in moderation and does not lead from the low sugar curve into the high sugar.

We (Sapen sisters) act in a similar way. If we notice our glucose dropping gradually, we will consume 5-10 grams (g) of glucose, e.g. a few strawberries/grapes, one starburst, or one handful of popcorn.

It is important that you always keep in mind that 1 bread unit (BU) corresponds to approx. 10-12 g carbohydrates (carbs). To get out of your hypoglycemia we recommend the following carbohydrates supply:

BG 60-70 mg/dL = 10-12 carbs (1 BU)

BG 50-60 mg glucose level = 20-25 carbs (2 BU)

BG below 40 mg = 30-45 carbs (3-4 BU)

My personal tip:

Treating with the average of 20-25 carbs (2 BU) you aren't doing anything wrong and won't do harm- especially if you feel you have to act quickly.

What you should always have in your house:

- Direct juice or juice concentrate containing a minimum of 15 g carbs per serving

- Dextrose (2-3 tablets correspond to 8-12 g carbs = 1 BU)

- Fruit gummies (6 Haribo gold-bears correspond to approximately 10 carbs = 1 BU)

- Bananas (depending on the size, bananas may differ between 15-30 g carbs = 1 - 2 BU)

- Other fruit (e.g. grapes are approximately 1 g carb per piece, 10 grapes = 1 BU)

For on the road:

Small juice boxes or bottles from the supermarkets are great. These are available in the size of 12 to 16 ounces and the bottles can be closed again. We (Ashley and Emily) typically use the Apple & Eve 10 ounce resealable bottles. One bottle contains 30 g carbs and can be saved if only half is necessary at the time.

If you only have a smaller bag with you, some dextrose tablets, a few of the small Haribo gummies, or fun size Skittle packs will fit. One packet corresponds pretty much to 10 carbs/1 BU.

CHAPTER 9
DIETARY CHANGE

I (Vivi) have often thought that diabetes may have saved my life more than endangered it. When does a supposedly healthy person go to the doctor? We diabetics go to the practice every quarter. From blood to urine, eyes to heart, and weight to well-being, everything is checked, documented, and questioned.

As a diabetic - regardless of type - a healthy, nutritious diet is always recommended. That does not mean exclusively that one should lose weight with it. Rather, it is a matter of changing lifestyles, which may need to be turned upside down in order to reconsider "bad habits" and avoid long-term consequential damage.

We all find this topic very exciting. Also we fight again and again with our weight like many others. In fact, body weight also directly influences the amount of insulin necessary per unit of carbohydrate. We continuously keep an eye on what we are eating, love to try out new recipes and diets of all kinds to see how it affects our sugar levels, and try not to gain or lose too much weight.

In the following paragraph, Vivi explains how it worked for her until her last pregnancy. Were you aware that insulin is also an anabolic drug? This means that you gain weight if you take "too much" of it.

During pregnancy, my insulin requirement increased up to 270%. It was a vicious circle and for the first time I realized what insulin resistance was and the effect insulin played, as an anabolic agent, on my body and on my child. I ended up with a height of 177cm (5'9") and weighed 96 kg (211 lbs) and my child was born "macrosomia" (very tall and heavy). Already during pregnancy I was intensively occupied with various nutritional possibilities. As a diabetic, however, it had to be "diet hacks" to save calories but still give me enough energy to avoid many hypoglycemia events.

The following tips are suitable for anyone who wants a healthy diet. Those of you who want to lose weight should also make use of these tricks.

- Try to familiarize yourself with and use units of measurement. For example, measure the amount of spread used (1 teaspoon/tablespoon) per piece of bread.

Toppings and cooking alternatives

- Use fresh cheese and margarine as an alternative to butter. Light and low-fat products are recommended and even "double cream" of fresh cheese has 60% less fat and calories than butter.

- Use cream alternatives such as cream cheese and coconut milk. If you have fried meat, add one tablespoon (tbsp) of cream cheese or 1 tbsp of light coconut milk to your pan or roaster. They can be used to make excellent sauces that are just as tasty.

- In soups, finely grated potatoes or mashed potatoes are also excellent as a creamy binding agent.

- Leave the breadcrumbs, flour, and oil in the cupboard! Chop hazelnuts crumbly (preferably with a food processor) and use them as an alternative. You don't need any more flour either. Simply dip into egg yolk, then into hazelnut splinters and put directly into the oven with usually ~ 20 minutes at 400° Fahrenheit.

- Alternatively, eat meat simply in "nature" again and again.

- For cooking, use water instead of oil or use only 1 tsp to 1 tbsp of oil.

- For oven vegetables or meat: put everything in a pot, season it, and use 1 teaspoon of oil again. Then stir it with your hands in the pot before spreading onto the baking tray.

- If there is too little oil in the pan or on the tray, you can alternatively add water without any loss of taste!

The carbohydrate choice

- There are various alternatives to wheat flour noodles - potatoes, quinoa, bulgur & couscous - that contain less carbohydrates per serving.

- Noodles taste great, but they increase your appetite and you "can't get enough." The great alternatives are rice noodles (less than half the carbohydrates, but just as tasty) or ZUCCHINI noodles! (Just make sure that these are cooked after a few minutes! Zucchini noodles (also known as zoodles) can go a long away and taste great!

- As always, potatoes in all varieties, rice, quinoa, bulgur, couscous and millet are very tasty and filling.

- Spaghetti squash is a low-carb alternative to a plate of spaghetti. Top it with your favorite tomato sauce!

Choice of meat

- Pork is incredibly rich in calories and high in unhealthy fat. Try to switch to other types of meat whenever possible. Poultry meat is particularly recommended. Apply this idea:

Better without skin!

- For minced meat, I (Vivi) recommend minced beef or tartar. The latter is expensive, which is why I buy it less often. Aldi has minced beef with 70% less fat - a very good choice.

- When slicing, I also recommend choosing any kind of poultry slices, raw ham (with small or no fat edges), or fish! For example, stremel salmon, prawns, shrimps, trout, roll mops and mackerel are especially great. Fish provides you with healthy omega 3 fats, less caloric intake, and satiation.

- We (Ashley and Emily) are big into vegetable, quinoa, and even sweet potato burgers. We also choose to eat more chicken, ground turkey, and turkey patties rather than beef and pork.

Oven or steam cook rather than sear

- Browning is only possible with oil, therefore the oven is an excellent alternative.

- Most meat and fish dishes are best served with good seasoning, fresh herbs, and 1 tablespoon of oil. For a gentle way of cooking it is recommended to choose a steam cooker - especially for vegetables or spinach. The vegetables are steamed, contain all the vitamins, and remain sensationally crunchy.

RECIPE PROPOSAL:

Vegetables of your choice: e.g. quartered potatoes, carrots, broccoli, onions, zucchini, and eggplant.

Cut everything into small pieces and mix in a pot with 1 tsp olive oil.

- Spread generously on a baking tray.
- Mix 1 teaspoon of oil with ½ pressed lemon, pepper and salt and drizzle on one (or more) salmon fillets (instead of salmon you can also use a type of meat of your choice).
- Bake at 400°F for 20-25 minutes in the oven.

An alternative to flour and milk

Did you know that milk also has plenty of calories and is comparable to a small meal, even from a digestive point of view? For me (Vivi) this is super difficult, because I have always liked to drink coffee with milk my whole life.

Accordingly, I am now saving milk, along with flour, in other places. Where? For example with pancakes, muffins or cakes of all kinds. I substitute both flour and milk with oat flakes, egg, and banana.

RECIPE PROPOSAL:

Pancakes:

2	Bananas
1	Egg
4-5 tbsp.	Oat flakes
1 tsp.	baking powder

Puree everything and at the end - if you like - add blueberries. Heat only 1 teaspoon of oil in the pan. Drizzle small spoons with the pureed mixture onto your pan and bake on each side until golden brown - READY!

MUFFINS are similar: the basic mixture is always a squashed banana + egg + baking powder. You can also add cocoa powder or chocolate flakes, fruit or vegetables (e.g. carrots and apples with roses). After approximately 12 minutes in the oven at 350° F circulating air, your little cakes are ready!

Alternative pizza = tuna, cauliflower, or wraps

- Sometimes you just want junk food. Fortunately, there are low-calorie alternatives that are surprisingly tasty.

RECIPE PROPOSAL:

- Drain 1-2 cans of "tuna fish in water".

- Mix with an egg and puree as well.
- Spread the mixture on a baking tray lined with baking paper.
- Cover as you please.
- At 350°F circulating air in the oven - bake for about 10-15 minutes = time may vary depending on the ingredients you have placed on the pizza

The same can be done with cauliflower!

It is even easier to replace a pizza with wraps. Simply cover and enjoy in the oven after 10 minutes. Only tip: the bottom is softer here and can not be eaten quite as crispy as a pizza. But it is very tasty!

Buns for breakfast = it's all about sharing!

I love buns. But we all know how fast one has eaten one and that hunger often doesn't give in because appetite outstrips appetite. For this it is recommended to cut the bread roll like a baguette - into many slices. Then you have the possibility to take 4 to 5 slices out of one roll and can cover them differently. This way, more time is spent eating a single bread roll and you may become full more easily.

Dressing substitutes

- Yogurt dressing tastes just as good if not better than mayo and sometimes has over 70% (and more) less calories and fat. We (Ashley and Emily) have used greek yogurt as a substitute to mix with tuna - it is just as tasty and healthier- containing less fat, more protein, and nutrients such as calcium and probiotics!

- In southern countries, lemon is very popular as a dressing. In Turkey, many people don't use anything else! Give it a try! It tastes fresh. Seasoned with 1 tsp honey, salt and pepper, 1 pinch of mustard, 1 teaspoon water and herbs is a dressing at least as tasty as with oil!!!

- Another dressing I (Emily) frequently use on my salads is apple cider vinegar. It contains no fat, only few calories, and nearly zero carbs, whereas other vinaigrettes and dressings include up to approximately 15 g fat, 150 calories, and 10 g carbs per serving. Apple cider vinegar may aide in weight loss, reduce cholesterol, and improve digestion.

Instead of pure alcohol = prefer spritzers

- Especially if it is more about "drinking along", spritzers such as wine spritzers and alcoholic seltzers are recommended. This quenches thirst, makes dosing and managing sugar levels easier, and has neither many calories nor carbohydrates.

Milk Alternatives

- Nut milks contain much fewer calories and carbs. They also include healthy fats and protein which increase satiety. We (Ashley and Emily) have been on an almond milk trend for the last several years. Other options include soy, cashew, and coconut milk. We found the unsweetened vanilla almond milk, with less than 1 g of carbs per serving, to have less effect on our blood sugars than a serving of normal (2%) milk. You may find yourself using almond milk as a coffee creamer (making it practically a zero carb drink), in your protein shakes, smoothies, or even as a mid-day or evening snack!

WHOLE 30

We (Ashley and Emily) have achieved great success with blood sugar control on a low-carb diet. We followed the "Whole 30" meal plan for one month- hence the 30. Basics of the diet: no added sugars, no processed foods, no grains, no legumes, no alcohol. Only whole fruits and vegetables, unprocessed meats, fish, nuts and seeds, some oils, eggs, and seasonings are permitted for the month. The less label and more natural, the better.

To determine insulin needs, we found ourselves using a food scale to calculate carbohydrates often. It was worth the few extra minutes as it strengthened carb counting accuracy and taught us much about appropriate portion sizes!

Some of the benefits we gained to participating in Whole 30 included: increased energy and mood, losing a few pounds, increased insulin sensitivity, taking less insulin, improved BG control, and lessening our craving for sweets and carbs. View our experience on our "Whole30" highlight on our Instagram page.

Recipes can be found online, especially on Instagram @Whole30 and @Whole30recipes, and hashtags #Whole30 and #Whole30recipes. Some of our favorite snacks/meals include:

- Sweet potato toast (topped with either almond butter for sweet or guacamole, tuna, and cucumber as a meal)
- Salad with protein (chicken/pork/tuna) and vegetables
- Avocado (smashed) with cucumber slices/ peppers/ sugar snap peas
- Mexican stuffed sweet potato (with chicken, tomatoes, jalapenos, salsa, onion, cilantro,

garlic, taco seasoning)
- Whole 30 Chipotle bowl
- Breakfast plate: two over easy eggs, half of a baby avocado, and sauteed vegetables (bell peppers, mushroom, scallions, tomatoes)
- Sweet potato chicken poppers
- Bananas or Honeycrisp apples with 1-2 tbsp almond butter
- Dressings: apple cider vinegar, olive oil, ghee, Whole 30 buffalo ranch

Manage ravenous hunger attacks
- My (Vivi's) deepest tip is to add psyllium husks to your routine. Take 1-2 teaspoons and dissolve them in a glass of water or mix them with your food. You should drink plenty of liquid. The psyllium seed shells swell and saturate. They stimulate intestinal activity and promote digestion.
- Furthermore, proteins generally help against the small ravenous hunger attacks... e.g. boiled eggs or low-fat cheese or skyr, a cultured dairy product, made with "flavor drops" and liquid sweetener. Skyr is available from many suppliers, including Amazon. Poultry cold cuts (pure) are also an option.

- For the sweet hunger we recommend fruit, freshly made fruit mousse, semolina porridge, and dark chocolate (from 70%).

- Other nutritious snacks: nuts mixed with cranberries, raisins, chopped figs or apricots (whatever you like)! But beware, nuts and dried fruits also have MANY calories and fat. Count 3-5 pieces approximately and chop them (like fruits) - very quickly you have "more mass" to fill up on and a delicious, concentration-promoting snack.

Track your Intake

A very important note: If you want to lose weight, you have to achieve a caloric deficit. In other words, you must take in less energy than you spend. Like a savings account, it's about saving calories and not wasting everything you have.

Download an app to help you count calories and determine your basic needs. MyFitness Pal is a user-friendly, tracker app we use from time to time and also use daily if strictly logging and when we "want to get back on track". This app allows you to track your food, exercise, weight, and water intake. You set a goal and timeframe in which you want to achieve that goal... and the app customizes the total amount of nutrients necessary to fit your needs to reach the goal. It gives you illustration via a pie graph of all macronutrients you have consumed in a day- which helps to carb count more accurately, visualize what nutrients are lacking, and realize how much of and what you may need to cut back.

We (Ashley and Emily) are more than happy to help guide you in navigating MyFitness Pal.

Furthermore, we have tried numerous famous diets (fad) and want to share our biggest takeaway. With a majority carbohydrates intake coming from whole foods (fruits, vegetables, pure meats, etc...), blood sugar spikes can be better controlled and the total amount of daily insulin can be reduced significantly, especially once your body becomes more sensitive to it. By cutting out added sugar whenever possible, our cravings have been minimized and so have the sugar spikes. It does take time and practice to figure out your adjusted insulin needs and to minimize low blood sugars, but you will be left with a feeling of accomplishment from the hard work and success (in more than one aspect).

Although we choose to generally eat healthy, we understand the importance of "everything in moderation" and to not eliminate any major food group, as all are necessary. It is okay to treat yourself... it keeps your mind "happy and healthy". A good friend and master in the field of nutrition shared the 80/20 diet with us. If you are compliant with your diet and eat clean 80% of the time, you should allow yourself to indulge in less healthy food without guilt for the remaining 20% of your food intake. We love this approach and remind ourselves of this since it closely fits into our lifestyle and diet preference.

CHAPTER 10

EXERCISING WITH T1D

When it comes to exercising, there are just a few extra steps an individual with type one diabetes must take. It is important to understand this piece: there is not one single method that works for everybody. Type one diabetes is unpredictable and most diabetics have multiple techniques to choose between and implement on a daily basis. As identical twins, even our insulin requirements and diabetes needs differ greatly. We will share our personal experiences and tips throughout this chapter.

Multiple factors affect your blood sugar on a daily basis let alone the extra effect exercise can play on one's blood glucose. As stress, illness, insulin delivery and pump malfunctions, lack of sleep, anaerobic exercise (weight lifting), and too little insulin cause a rise in blood sugar, factors such as aerobic exercise (cardio), too much insulin, and a diet lacking a balance of nutrients can cause a drop in blood sugar. Some individuals see a rise in blood sugar with exercise, most likely from the body's release of cortisol when adrenaline is present (weight-lifting). It is more common for us to experience hypoglycemia with exercise, as both our lifting and cardio/cross-training workouts are considered to be high intensity. Our lifts include short intervals of cardio between sets to keep our heart rates elevated, which also avoids a spike in our blood sugars.

Planning your exercise routine is essential, however it is not always realistic. In addition to the factors listed above, your level/intensity of activity from the previous 12 to 24 hours also plays a role in blood sugar.

You have to take into account the time of day and whether you plan to exercise upon awakening or post-work shift. More times than we can count, we do everything to prepare - eat a balanced snack or meal, decrease our basal insulin, and begin the workout with a sugar in range - and our BGs still drop without reason.

On top of trying to stay fit and in good health, it certainly is a challenge adding in the management of diabetes with exercise. We were actively involved in extracurricular sports and activities through grade school and college... and still are! Instead of viewing it as a struggle or excuse to skip exercising, we take it as another daily challenge. Challenge accepted!

The Twins' Tips and Tricks to Working Out:

Don't give up! Figuring out what works best to keep your sugars from spiking or falling takes time. Throughout the past few years we have come up with multiple methods and still they do not always work according to plan.

Each day may bring different factors, so listen to your body and blood sugar. Try the method that you feel is best and see if it works for you! If it does, write it down. If it doesn't, still write it down. Try it on a different day and maybe it will work in a different situation.

Create a list of patterns you experience before, during, and after exercise. This is helpful for comparing workout days after work vs before work, day shift vs night shift, and morning vs night.

Try setting a temporary basal rate at a decreased or increased rate. Start low. (30-50% less for half an hour) We have found that setting them an hour prior to working out works best for us for high-intensity exercise. However, planning is key to be able to set these in advance. When possible to try setting a temporary basal, go for it!

Keep quick-acting sugar (e.g. juice, glucose tabs, candy) on hand while working out or at least be quickly accessible in the locker room!

Wear a medical alert! It is best to be fully prepared in case you were to run into an emergency, especially if alone. We would hope a first responder would recognize the medic alert on our wrist if we were unconscious.

If you ever have any questions about exercising and T1D, whether it deals with sports or working out in general, feel free to reach out at any time! You may contact us via email or our social media platforms (Instagram and Facebook) and we will be more than happy to support and assist you!

CHAPTER 11

TYPE ONE DIABETES IN PREGNANCY

As Ashley and Emily have not yet experienced diabetes and pregnancy, the following chapter content includes Vivi's experiences and advice.

Just 40 years ago, type 1 diabetics were advised against getting pregnant and giving birth to children. At that time it was not known exactly why the mortality and disability rate among diabetic children was so high, but even without scientific evidence at the time it was certain that diabetes was the cause. The doctors agreed that the greatest risk for pregnant diabetics was high blood sugar. Until more than 35 years ago, however, stable blood sugar could not be properly controlled or permanently stabilized.

There is no doubt that insulins were not as developed as they are today. Long-acting insulins did not yet exist, neither insulin pens nor insulin pumps, nothing had been tested for pregnancy, and the suspected risks had been scientifically proven. In the 1970s Rolf Renner, among others, used small injection-perfusion for the first time in France and Germany to introduce insulin into a vein. This was the beginning of insulin pumps.

Sensors that can measure blood sugar were created. Blood sugar monitoring sensors such as today's "Freestyle Libre" or the continuous glucose monitor sensor created by Dexcom were still the absolute dream of the future.

This new method of BG management is excellent compared to the common diabetes therapy, but there were major problems with the access route. Since it is basically an infusion of insulin, a venous cannula had to be inserted. In addition, inflammation of the peripheral blood vessels occurred regularly. At the end of the 1970s, working groups in Great Britain and Germany under Renner, Walter, Sonnenberg and Chantelau began infusing into the subcutaneous fatty tissue, thus laying the foundation for the "continuous subcutaneous insulin infusion" which is still common today. However, the first pumps to be used were not insulin pumps in the true sense of the word. These were small, motor-driven devices that were used, among other things, for pain therapy. The delivery rates of these devices were not calibrated for insulin units, i.e. the units had to be converted each time in a time-consuming manner.

All in all, having diabetes was much more of a burden back then. The disease alone led directly to a lower life expectancy. Late effects of diabetes and complications were common. As a diabetic woman, one was ultimately exposed to very high risks during pregnancy, without the doctors being able to do much for her at that time. In addition, relationships often broke down due to a strong, unfulfilled desire to have children. But it is even worse if you lose a child due to illness or if he or she suffers disabilities as a result. These issues were everyday mental burdens for many type 1 diabetics almost 40 years ago.

Fortunately, we type 1 diabetics can now become pregnant just as easily and healthily as any other woman. There is an average inheritance risk of only 5%. Although this is the case, type 1 diabetics are still advised against spontaneous, unplanned pregnancies. The pregnancy of diabetics is still risky and should therefore begin with controlled, stable blood sugar levels. It is recommended that the woman has Hgb A1C of 7% mmol or less before conception.

To date, there is minimal literature on the changing insulin requirement during pregnancy for type 1 diabetics. My endocrinologist explained that this is partly due to the fact that the rise in blood sugar and increased insulin requirements are also related to the progress of the pregnancy and growth of the baby. She concluded that there was still too little research in this area.

Now that I have already had two pregnancies, I would like to share my most important experiences with you.

1. Try to obtain a HgbA1C between 6 and 7 mmol before conception.

2. Once you have pregnancy plans, take folic acid. It is suggested that the stronger preparation (4-5mg/day) does the most good for diabetics.

3. Pay attention to your iron values from the beginning. It becomes critical in the middle of pregnancy. If you provide an iron-rich meal right from the start, you may prevent this possibility from occurring.

4. Do a toxoplasmosis test. This will test your blood for antibodies to certain parasites, possibly transmitted by contact with cats or consumption of red meat.

5. You should also have a test done for chlamydia and cytomegaly. These viruses are usually not noticed automatically, but can lead to various complications during pregnancy including underdevelopment and miscarriages.

6. Be in physical top form if you want to get pregnant. I'm alluding to your weight.

7. Keep a diary for 3 months so that you are quickly equipped with an insulin pump and a blood sugar monitoring log, preferably during the first weeks of pregnancy!

8. Fight cravings and the ravenous appetite. Get used to low-sugar desserts right from the start and limit the number per day. The best thing is to bake it yourself. Weight Watchers recipes are great.

9. Orient yourself on your diet and the kitchen - Weight Watchers recipes are really varied, balanced and tasty. You should not under any circumstances diet during pregnancy, but don't let yourself go!

10. Don't consume too many carbohydrates! The insulin requirement for a woman and her infant rises strongly from about the 5th month of pregnancy onwards.

At the end of my pregnancy, I had 270% of my insulin needs, which is exceptionally high. According to my endocrinologist, the vast majority of type 1 diabetics seem to rise to about 200%. But that means that you have to inject yourself accordingly (twice the amount) for all carbohydrates.

Don't forget: INSULIN IS AN ANABOLIC DRUG. The more insulin you ingest, the more likely you are to gain weight and the more likely it is that your child will become macrosomic (very large and heavy)! Macrosomia also increases the risk of type two diabetes in the infant.

11. Exercise regularly during pregnancy! If necessary, have your working hours reduced. It is important that you promote your health to the maximum. Diabetes itself makes pregnancy sufficiently difficult. I recommend walking or swimming.

12. Ask for a gynecologist with experience in type 1 diabetes (not gestational diabetes!).

13. A prenatal class may be offered to diabetics free of charge. You should take note of this in order to have all risks clarified in the long term (there are also sensational ultrasound images).

14. Choose a hospital for delivery with an affiliated children's hospital. If anything goes wrong due to diabetes, you AND YOUR CHILD are best looked after here.

Draw attention to your diabetes several times when registering at the hospital. After childbirth, you lose weight quickly and insulin requirements decrease immediately. The risk of hypoglycemia is immediate. In my experience, it seemed that everyone took care of my child, but no one took care of me. The nurses completely underestimated the severity of type 1 diabetes. Therefore: Take bananas, gummy bears, and juice with you so that you can help yourself if necessary!

It is a fact that with close medical care and much discipline, pregnancy can be well managed and a healthy child can be developed in the body and born. Nevertheless, there may be a few "black" moments full of panic - sometimes due to severe hypoglycemia and then with ketoacidosis. This is caused by the fluctuating insulin requirement which, as I mentioned, increases continuously during pregnancy.

My endocrinologist calmed me down and accompanied me from the time of my pregnancy plans and well into the breastfeeding period. I was in such luck that my endocrinologist gave me her mobile phone number and was also available via "What's App" - day and night. At first I thought that this offer was friendly, but I wouldn't take advantage. This attitude quickly changed because the sudden responsibility for another life, depending on you, makes a woman very sensitive and anxious.

There is no doubt that this phase of life also has many double burdens for type 1 diabetics and in many respects it is a true test!

I will summarize all preparation points as a checklist for you as follows:

At least 3 months BEFORE pregnancy:

- Hgb A1c between 6 and 7
- Pay attention to your figure
- Keep a diabetes diary
- Take folic acid
- Check blood values (take iron if necessary)
- Refresh vaccinations
- Consider toxoplasmosis test
- Get tested for chlamydia & cytomegaly
- Search for a gynecologist with diabetes experience

Beginning of pregnancy:

- Search for a midwife (immediately after the 12th week is finished!)
- Ask for the mobile phone numbers of your doctors (especially endocrinologists)
- Hospital search with endocrinologists and a children's hospital
- Apply for insulin pump (if you do not already have)

- Address your own situation in the hospital and be sure the system creates a medical record.
- Get keto strips at the pharmacy (be sure to have them in stock at home!)
- Exercise regularly
- Pay attention to carbohydrates (try to keep between 150-250 carbohydrates per day (15-20 BUs)

After childbirth

- Expect hypoglycemia and be prepared. Take a lot of fast-acting sugar with you to the hospital.
- Overcome your pain and BREASTFEED! It is the best preventive measure for your child to develop diabetes itself.

I (Emily) am a postpartum maternity nurse. I was very disappointed to hear Vivi's personal experience of feeling that her management of diabetes was underestimated after birth. The biggest piece of advice I can give from my perspective is to speak with your nurses and keep them up to date. You are going through so much both during and after childbirth that you should be able to depend on the help from your nurses.

Work experience has taught me that patients with type one may choose to do one of two things for in the hospital: you may set a plan with your obstetric group prior to hospitalization to either be independent with your diabetes management or use the help provided by your doctor and healthcare team (in which there will be pre-set orders the nurse will follow to manage your diabetes: BG checks, sliding scale for coverage, etc.). The choice may be up to you and your obstetric group.

It is critical to inform your nurse if you are nervous or concerned about your blood sugar in the midst of everything else going on. We practice couplet care, meaning we take quality care of both MOM and BABY. Your health is just as important as your child's! It is a special night at work when I care for a type one diabetic as I truly enjoy caring for, connecting with, and learning from them. If a patient with type one is under the care of another nurse, I do everything I can to support both the nurse and the patient. I make myself an available resource in case a coworker needs my input, knowledge, or experience. It is not surprising to me that questions arise because the occurrence of caring for a patient with type one happens seldomly.

As I have not yet experienced motherhood, I attempt to make every interaction I have with a type one patient a learning experience. I plan to build on my knowledge throughout these experiences to be best prepared (to care for future patients with type one and myself).

CHAPTER 12

INSULIN PUMP VERSUS PEN

During pregnancy and lactation it is recommended to switch to an insulin pump and a blood sugar sensor if you are not already using them.

Applying for the equipment is complex because it is very expensive. Not every diabetic has the possibility to change supplies under normal conditions with decent blood sugar values and the support of the health insurance.

As a pregnant woman in Germany, it is virtually "self-run". No pregnant woman may be rejected the equipment. Once you have the equipment, you may extend the loan of the equipment again and again even after breastfeeding.

Until my pregnancy, I had an insulin pen for over 12 years and was managed very well with a combination of Lantus, Metformin, and NovoRapid. I personally found it annoying to suddenly sit down on a catheter from a pump site and permanently "store" a "device" on my body. Now, however, I have to admit that my average blood sugar values became constant with the help of the insulin pump (= 6.0 mmol)!

When using the insulin pump, only one type of insulin, usually fast-acting, is infused continuously over 24 hours (in small, various doses). This makes it possible to completely imitate the function of a pancreas. This is especially important at night, when the cortisol level rises irregularly, a different dosage can be set every hour. Throughout the day, different "basal" patterns can be set for each hour. The basal rate is the amount of insulin that is infusing continuously. So, if one notices that they are generally running higher blood sugars in the afternoon, their basal rate can be set to administer a higher, more precise insulin dosage over that time period.

With the insulin pump it is even possible to inject incredibly small doses of 0.05 of a unit, allowing a precision of insulin therapy that simply cannot be imitated with regular insulin pens.

After my first pregnancy, I (Vivi) decided the only option was to return to my old pen system of multiple daily injections. I accepted that my Hgb A1C values would get worse again. Today - after my second pregnancy - I decided in favor of the pump and the blood sugar sensor. Since my blood sugar values are by far better with the pump - above all also in difficult and/or changeable life phases (little sleep and bright nerves) - I undertake something with receipt of my pump. In my opinion, the insulin pump will decrease my chances of later complications and even lengthen my lifespan.

The discussion of insulin pen versus insulin pump, however, is still an exciting one. I didn't make the decision easy for myself because carrying a pump on your body is simply a bigger and more visible obstacle than carrying an insulin pen invisibly in your pocket.

Read our comparative analysis between insulin pen and insulin pump below:

PEN	**PUMP**
With the help of a coordinated basal and bolus therapy one tries to cover 24 hours of insulin supply.	Precise adjustment of the insulin dosage over 24 hours with only one insulin.
Insulin delivery is possible from increments 0.5 Units.	Insulin doses may vary from 0.05 of a unit.
You must adhere to the office hours or opening hours of your doctors and pharmacies.	24-hour service from the pump manufacturer.

PEN	PUMP
You will receive all the aids for a pen in the pharmacy - often also from your doctor, who has many samples in stock from the pharmaceutical representatives.	With the exception of the plasters, you can only obtain aids through the direct sales of the pharmaceutical company of your pump.

Clearly arranged aids that are easy to store, take with you and stow away:	Unbelievably many aids that have to be stowed away and when you are on the road (business trips or vacation), this means thinking about packing a lot and accordingly:
- Basal/bolus pen or insulin vial - Needle caps - Alcohol swabs - Insulin cartridges One drawer for the utensils is sufficient.	- Catheters/infusion sets - Tubing (if applicable) - Insulin vial - Batteries - Possibly insulin pockets or clips - Pump - Pump site adhesives You will need one half of the cabinet or at least 3 drawers to accommodate all the aids.
PEN	**PUMP**
With the pen, always check that the syringe head is free before injecting - this is not possible with the pump, as	If the pump does not immediately notice a catheter issue, it may also be possible that you will not be supplied with

the catheter is in your body.	insulin for several hours.
In the US, your endocrinologist/doctor can provide you with a prescription to easily pick up your insulin vials or pens. In Germany, every diabetic with an intensified insulin therapy receives an injection set. Most doctors have a syringe in stock and can give it to you free of charge.	Complex application and approval of a pump by the health insurance companies. The application must be renewed regularly. The cost is much more.
Doctors and healthcare workers are experienced in dealing with all pens and insulins. In addition to the doctors, you can usually also ask the medical assistants or your endocrinologist or dietitian. (There is	Doctors and the healthcare team may not necessarily be familiar with the operation of your insulin pump - you will have to contact your representative or the manufacturer for specific questions.

therefore enough knowledged people to contact).	
PEN	**PUMP**
No unnoticed clogging possible.	The pump regularly and unexpectedly indicates a "clogging" and reports this with a beep of noise.
Nothing has to be changed at night and if necessary you can change and check all cartridges before going to bed.	It is not unusual for you to have to reconnect your complete pump system in the middle of the night due to an occlusion and/or pump malfunction.
A very good Hgb A1C can be achieved with syringe therapy if the diabetic himself understands his diabetes and the influencing factors. One must remember to take the long-acting insulin injection rather than the pump self-	The pump enables an excellent Hgb A1c. The basal rate can even be set as a percentage, e.g. hourly to 60% instead of 100% or increased to 140%. In difficult circumstances such as pregnancy, illness, etc., this is exceptionally great because you can carefully approach the fluctuating insulin

delivering a basal insulin.	requirements.
PEN	**PUMP**
With a pen you can only inject for your carbohydrate intake immediately. Should food be digested later or lead to an increase in blood sugar, this can only be regulated by additional measurement, observation, and corrective injections.	With a pump, you can determine the time intervals for insulin delivery. This becomes very interesting for foods that go slowly into the blood or have a low GI (glycemic index). (e.g. whole grain noodles, pizza, foods containing high fat content)
The pen is easy to use in any sport. Everything fits into a belly belt: pure sugar, blood sugar meter, and pen and needles - and off you go. When swimming, everything is in a bag within easy reach. When swimming with an insulin pump, one would have to disconnect and	The pump is unsuitable for sports, especially if you perspire heavily. The adhesive may not hold the catheter under the skin in case of a lot of sweat. You run the risk of the insulin supply being interrupted (possibly even unnoticed). You will also need a strong belt so that the pump (if it includes tubing and constant connection) does

miss insulin if the pump is not waterproof .	not wobble back and forth when you are jogging, for example.
	One usually disconnects the pump (and leaves the catheter in the body) for exercises of quick duration.
	For sports that require a longer time period, top athletes may insert several catheters so that at least one still functions afterwards.
No one may realize or guess you are diabetic if you are using a pen.	The catheter hangs out of you with a small tubing. (depending on the pump).
You don't have the syringe with you when you shower.	The pump that Ashley and Emily use is "wireless" and does not require tubing.
You feel normal. Everything you do, you may feel like a healthy person.	Depending on where you have placed the catheter, it can even hurt if the needle is stuck or inserted in your body by "counterpressure".
	The pump is visible. You

	always have something on your body that looks "abnormal" or even "morbid" to outsiders.
	When showering and bathing, you must always leave a part of yourself out and wash around the catheter or disconnect and possibly miss basal insulin.
	You often have to answer questions and talk about your diabetes.
PEN	**PUMP**
Holiday, sun, & wellness of any kind do not bother your pen. Replacement is easy to get and packed, cooling bags are also available in slim sizes, and these are practical for all kinds of vacations.	Apart from the many aids you have to take with you, a catheter with a transfer tube may not withstand the sun, heat, salt water or even saunas for long on vacation. (You should pack "double and triple" extra aids)
	It is typical to have a backup emergency pen or insulin vial too.

Whether dresses, tight waistcoats, slim-fit blouses or jeans - with or without pockets... You can wear whatever you want with a pen system because your diabetes utensils are in your handbag rather than attached to your body.	Pump manufacturers have various belts and bags to stow the palm-sized pump on your body.
	Meanwhile, young enterprises discovered a market in it. The company "Ruby Limes" produces underpants with an integrated insulin pump pocket. The company "Hid in" has designed leg straps and other alternative fastening straps to accommodate the insulin pump beautifully and as inconspicuous as possible on the body.
	The pump often fits in trouser pockets - one of the simplest, most practical and free solutions.
With a pen you are stopped to inject at a distance of at least 5 cm to your navel. In addition,	The catheter of a pump is worn on the body for an average 2-3 days. This may leave areas of redness and

you should use a different injection site with every stick to avoid nodules, hardening, or inflammation. Previous injection sites are hardly found because the needle is tiny.	skin irritation due to the catheter patch and the sticker that is over it.
To inject, you always have to uncover a part of the body, The abdomen and leg are fast and rarely noticed. However in fine or strange company, it is better to go to the restroom.	You can bolus completely unnoticed on the pump. This is either via Bluetooth control or manually directly on the pump. Ignorant people have no idea what kind of device it is and may not see that it is connected to our body.
When you go to sleep, put your diabetic test bag on the bedside table. It has everything you need in case of an emergency. While sleeping, you don't need these utensils.	If on a pump with tubing, you can wear the pump on a belt while sleeping or let it fall loosely next to you in bed or stow the pump in your underpants. If you don't move much during the night, that's no problem. Otherwise it may happen that you get

	tangled up in your own tubing, lie down on your pump, or that it falls off your bed and painfully "rips" the catheter out of your body.

You can see how complex this topic is!

In spite of all my criticism, I (Vivi) chose the insulin pump. The risk reduction of late effects and complications with the help of the excellent blood sugar values are - in my opinion - definitely worth it.

Furthermore, I even believe that every diabetic should be allowed to try out this system for 6 - 12 months. The reduction of late effects can actually be in the interest of the health insurance company. Find a doctor who will support you argumentatively in your application.

Another important hint:

Today's insulin pumps also have bluetooth. This allows the user to connect the pump to a matching glucometer. With the help of this measuring device you can inject an insulin dose unnoticed publicly without having to pull the pump out of your pocket. This solution is also suitable for small children with type 1. For children, a pump is certainly more attractive. The catheter is changed about 2-3 times a week, eliminating the need for constant injections during the day. In addition, parents can take over the insulin dosage of their children unnoticed using the aforementioned bluetooth technology.

Whichever one chooses, they may be well controlled. It is all dependent on how one manages their diabetes best, which fits their lifestyle, and which they will enjoy most.

We (the Sapen sisters) were fortunate to have the opportunity to start on insulin pumps shortly after diagnosis- at age 8. We LOVED our Medtronic insulin pumps and had the most fashionable "pump pouches" to match our daily outfits and cheerleading uniforms.

We then took a break from pump therapy during our high school years. Throughout high school, we were getting tired of the idea of "being connected" to the tubing and the pump 24/7. At the time, it was an annoyance to find somewhere to hold our pump on every piece of clothing we picked out. In addition, we were very active participating in after school activities such as lacrosse, dance, tumbling, and cheerleading. We would find ourselves disconnecting from our pumps so often to prevent them from being dislodged. We wanted a change.

With this being said, we went back to taking multiple daily injections for several years and were managing decently in relation to the many factors of "growing up". It worked for us, especially while cheering on a collegiate team.

Halfway through college, we spoke with our healthcare provider about the current possible treatment options. We decided to try insulin pumps again. Since we first stopped using a pump, the Omnipod pump became available. This pump is "tubeless", meaning that no pump tubing is involved from the pump itself to the infusion site. The Omnipod system also works wirelessly from the PDM (meter/pump control system) to the pod (infusion site on the body). The infusion site is larger in comparison to other pump sites/catheters since the insulin is included and held right there... however it is simply amazing!

There are many options available now to manage type one. There is also so much more to come with the ongoing advancements in technology. It is inspiring that diabetics have OPTIONS which are comparable in quality to suit their personal needs! We suspect that within the next 10 years, maybe even sooner, treatment options will advance drastically.

CHAPTER 13

GROWING UP WITH T1D IN SCHOOL

SINCE WE (ASHLEY AND EMILY) WERE DIAGNOSED AT A YOUNGER AGE, WE WOULD LIKE TO SHARE SOME EXPERIENCES AND TIPS FOR THE YOUNG INDIVIDUALS GROWING UP WITH DIABETES.

It is important to set up a meeting with your school nurse prior to the school year or within the first week of school, especially if it is a new school or nurse handling one's diabetic needs and treatment.

Elementary School

Since you/your child will have one primary teacher each year of grade school, it would be a good idea to have a meeting with the diabetic, mother/father, school nurse, and teacher (at the minimum). This will ease some nervousness/stress for all. Topics to cover include: when to go to the nurse's office, symptoms of low blood sugar, what to do in the event of a school or classroom party, bathroom breaks/possible frequency, being escorted by a friend or responsible person to the nurse if needed, and most importantly how to handle an emergency situation. We were always very fortunate to have knowledgeable and kind teachers that were willing to learn. We hope everyone would be provided with the same situation. Some teachers even kept a "goodie bag" of "low snacks" in the cabinet labeled with our names. Although the classrooms were not located too far from the nurse's office and one with hypoglycemia would be heading there anyway, it is reassuring to have sugar available for the "what if" situations.

Middle School
Prepare

In most middle schools, the school day is split between several teachers or a team of teachers. This means that there would be many more teachers/staff caring for the diabetic. It is just as important, if not more important, to set up a meeting with all teachers involved and discuss the basics of type one diabetes. In the ideal case, teachers would appreciate the initiative to increase awareness and safety. These teachers are also spending only brief periods throughout the school day with the student so a refresher of the key points here and there would be beneficial.

To reiterate, the following points should be addressed:

- Symptoms of hypoglycemia and hyperglycemia
- Hypoglycemia treatment/protocol (may be specific for one but certainly involves going to the nurse's office)
- The need to stay hydrated in times of hyperglycemia
- The need to frequently empty the bladder with hyperglycemia
- The need for someone to escort the diabetic to the nurse (for safety)
- The alarms that may sound during class (some of them you cannot turn off) and one may have to pull out their insulin pump or device to silence it or

Any additional information specific to the student and how he/she cares for themselves

At some point throughout middle school, perhaps the student will have the opportunity to gain some responsibility. This is a discussion that the diabetic and/or family would have to discuss with the teacher, nurse, faculty, and most likely the healthcare provider.

An example of gaining more responsibility during school hours may be having the privilege to carry your own meter and glucose testing supplies on hand. In our experiences, insulin has always (and we feel should always) be kept in the nurse's office. This is for medication safety: for the diabetic, staff, and other students. Also, the student should take a trip/stop by the nurse's office with abnormal blood sugars and at lunch time. Having the little bit of freedom of carrying some supplies teaches one to keep track of necessities and to begin gaining more independence of caring for themselves. Another possibility to work up to may be to stop in the nurse's office between classes (on the way to lunch or before the last class period) instead of missing a few minutes of either. These few changes really made a difference when we were given the opportunity. A safety risk is involved with both of these, however, and that must always be kept in mind. In addition, these opportunities are a privilege. If they are taken advantage of, they can be taken away at any time and it is important to reinforce that fact.

High School

Gaining Responsibility

If a diabetic is able to and can prove they are responsible, the same option of carrying supplies on hand may be possible throughout high school. The same considerations apply for one to carry his/her own equipment safely. A contract should be made with strict rules and regulations.

Follow your heart

As explained above, in high school the Sapen sisters wished for a "break" from their insulin pumps. After being "hooked up" with tubing for 7+ years, they wanted a change. This was one of those times where we were old enough to make advised decisions for ourselves, and so we went back to multiple daily injections. Looking back, it was one of the best things we chose to do. Thankfully, our overall management of our conditions were not much different between the two types of therapies. However, it switched up our daily routine for a couple years. As you may know, the corporation Omnipod has a wireless communicating insulin pump system. This was the perfect fit for us at the time and we still could not be happier with the decision to try it. The key point we would like to focus on about this is to speak up, keep your mind open to options, and use your educator and endocrinologist for advice. There are options and whichever makes you happiest and well controlled is best.

Obtaining a Driver's License

Depending on the state in which one resides, it is most likely that one will try to obtain their driver's license during their high school years. At your diabetes check ups around that time, have a talk with your healthcare provider. They or your parents may have specific suggestions or requirements for you when wanting your license. Some of the specific "rules" that we created together with our parents and endo include:

- Checking your blood glucose before sitting behind the wheel
- If your blood glucose is lower than 80 mg/dL or trending downwards towards a low glucose, you may not drive until the BG is treated and rechecked
- Always keep low supplies handy and fully stocked in the car (some examples include juice boxes, Skittles, gummies, and glucose tablets)
- Keep extra supplies (at least 1 box of strips, pump/MDI supplies, glucagon emergency kit, syringes, etc.)
- Wear a medical alert identification

Extracurricular Activities

The most crucial point we can stress to you about participating in extracurricular activities (e.g. sports, school activities) is being prepared. It is of utmost importance to have the necessary supplies on hand, whether it is kept in an after-school bag, at the nurse's or athletic trainer's office, or with the team's medical equipment. Have a meeting with the coaches and medical staff in charge prior to the sport season or start of the activity if going to be continued. Discuss with them the previously mentioned topics: the necessary accommodations/breaks, roles, and emergency situations.

College

The aspects of college have been scattered throughout the book between Vivi's experiences and also ours. The main topics include handling management of blood glucose during stress, partying, waking up to blood glucose alarms, and managing your diabetes on your own. Having a support friend, or several of them, is extremely helpful in all of the new and different experiences and people you are meeting, during classes and trips, in the dormitory building, party situations, and many other circumstances you will understand as they occur. College itself is stressful, so try to minimize the stress of managing your diabetes.

CHAPTER 14

THE IMPORTANCE OF SUPPORT

SOCIAL MEDIA

The easiest and most simple way to connect with other T1Ds in this world is through social media. We encourage you to explore the support systems through Facebook and Instagram specifically. There are hundreds, probably thousands of pages created on Facebook labeled specifically for diabetics. Some are focused on certain insulin pumps, Dexcom or Libre CGMs, location of state/area, sports and exercise, support groups, pregnancy, recipes, and pretty much anything else you could dream or think of! Some page examples we are part of include "T1D Eastern/Central PA", "Omnipod Users", and "Type 1 Diabetic Athletes". Experiences are shared, questions are asked, friendships are created, tips and tricks are explained, success is celebrated, low times are guided, and one's support is confirmed.

Instagram is set up different, but the same support is tremendously shared between millions and millions of diabetics. As we created @DoubleTheInsulin and saw Vivi's @sugarbootcamp page, we were opened to the world of T1D on Instagram and are still amazed today. Instagram accounts are run by people uploading pictures, text, and videos, and explaining things you experience and question every single day. Not a day goes by that we do not learn a new piece of information or come across something remarkable. There are mothers of diabetics, siblings with diabetes, adults with T1D, people that don't know anyone else with diabetes, companies that have products to help people like us, and more whom we communicate with daily. We support others and gain just as much support back. The positives, negatives, truths we do not wish to believe, tips, and life experiences are all out there.

Finally, Youtube is another outlet for support through social media. We met a friend from Canada through a type one event that vlogs (does mainly video blogging) through Youtube. Her work is truly inspiring and we can see how helpful it is for others!

DIABETES CAMP

We (Ashley and Emily) were encouraged by others to attend a diabetic youth camp shortly after diagnosis. We went for the week-long sleep away camp that upcoming summer. We were eight years old. We attended each summer thereafter until age fifteen. From attending as campers to now volunteering, we look forward to this week more than ever. We experienced the camping prospective, lived the counselor aspect, and now also attended as medical staff. Kids learn so much at camp. They learn information to live better medically, how to count carbohydrates, how their insulin works and dosing for each meal, and very important: that they are not alone. They try new insulin pump sites, an injection by themselves, an insulin site change independently for the first time, and gain confidence and independence in managing their condition. These children are truly inspiring and helpful to one another. This huge support system and group of people they can relate to is like a second family. Everyone we have met over the years hold a special place in our hearts. Some of life's best memories are from diabetes camp. Since age eight, it has always been "the best week of the year". Our hope is that every diabetic can attend a camp such as this one once in their life.

CHAPTER 15

ASHLEY AND EMILY'S LAST WORDS OF ADVICE

GLUCAGON: A Life-saving Measure

One of the most important things to learn about regarding diabetes is the administration of glucagon. This topic was covered previously, however we would like to emphasize the importance. When appropriate, it is vital to teach family, friends, the school nurse, coaches, parents, coworkers, and others what the glucagon is and how to use it.

After teaching the administration of glucagon and one explains their understanding, it is just as vital to PRACTICE the steps. As many can attest, learning is different from practicing, and practicing is VERY different than a real situation. It is beneficial for all to feel comfortable practicing the administration of the life-saving drug. The process may not be as clear in an emergency situation.

Although no one wants to feel confident in doing this for the fact that it is sincerely "a scary situation" it is essential.

LOGGING

A quick but also key in keeping a tight control of blood sugar values and management is logging. By keeping track of times, blood sugars, food (correct carbs, protein, fats), exercise, and other factors of the day, patterns become SO clear. Ashley and Emily logged their statistics in "The Diabetic Health Journal" (as shown on their social media account). After just two months of certain logging, both had a decrease in their HgbA1C by 0.7% mmol! The specific logging book has a "Decide and Conquer Diabetes Tribe" Facebook page to encourage and support the healthy habit!

EXTRA EXTRA

A piece of advice that will be so important to keep in mind is "always have extra supplies". Although you pack enough insulin, testing strips, batteries, and additional supplies for even a night away, you should have back up for the extra supplies! We have been caught more times than once running out of the extra supplies. Accidents, coincidences, bad absorption, and sick days happen. Always be prepared!!

GREATER THAN THE HIGHS AND LOWS

We live by the motto: "I am greater than my highs and lows". Crazy enough, we came across it through social media a couple years ago. We "preach" this motto by explaining it whenever given the chance. For many situations, but specifically type one diabetics, strength comes from within. One is thrown high points (literally and figuratively) and low points in life, and you are stronger than them! You cannot let them define you. You must find the courage from within to continue your fight through the tough times. Learn from the lows and celebrate the highs. We practice what we preach and truly believe this is an important guide in our daily lives.

STAY INVOLVED

However you wish, we hope that you choose to stay involved and connected with others living with and organizations supporting T1D. Whether it is your local JDRF (Juvenile Diabetes Research Foundation) chapter, online community, fundraising walks, or video blogs, stay connected! It is a way to continue learning, about diabetes, yourself, and your future.

We have come across countless opportunities and experiences that arose from our connections and organizations. There have been events and once in a lifetime opportunities we were fortunate to take part in! The people you connect with will make a difference in your life. In some ways, living with type one diabetes has made our lives better. We are strong. You are all so strong. So live your life without limits.

CLOSING WORD

This first book has hopefully given you a good introduction to the world of diabetes.

With the help of the content provided, you should now be able to distinguish between the different types of diabetes.

In addition, you have gained sound knowledge about how to communicate your diabetes to the outside world and which (communicative) strengths can be developed through the disease in your environment.

This book has been able to give you information on how to find the most suitable career as a type 1 diabetic. In addition, we have shown you how to deal with a chronic disease such as type 1 diabetes in all the "ups and downs" of your career.

In this context, I (Vivi) also briefly dealt with sensitive topics such as applying for a severely disabled person's card. This will hopefully help simplify your decision making and show you where you can go to apply in order to keep your own efforts to a minimum.

Furthermore, the book has prepared you in detail for stays abroad - whether short or long - excellent and provided you with many useful tips.

The book also covers topics such as parties,

alcohol and drugs, and diets with helpful tips on changing your diet.

The preparation and the course of a pregnancy with type 1 was presented as well as a comparison analysis between insulin pen and insulin pump, which should help you in your decision making.

Furthermore, the Sapen Sisters discussed experience and tips to best manage type one diabetes throughout school-age years.

In our opinion, the most elementary topics for young people have been addressed and dealt with.

For more in-depth questions or assistance, we are here to help.

We (Ashley and Emily) make ourselves available through our Facebook and Instagram messaging and email, @doubletheinsulin@gmail.com.

I (Vivi) offer you the opportunity to take advantage of my

"Sugar Mentoring". Whether per single hour via Skype or What's App, in a workshop (from 3 persons) or as a half-day or full-day seminar. See more details on my website www.sugarbootcamp.com and feel free to contact me anytime by e-mail: in-fo@sugarbootcamp.com

Further books will be published in 2019, which will supplement the contents of this copy. In the first quarter of 2019, for example, a book on "Taboo Topics in the Diabetes World" will be published.

Here, topics such as sexuality, obesity and emotional stress (stress, anxiety, depression and grief) find their place.

You can also look forward to online mentoring offers where I can personally take you by the hand and individually support you. In this context there will be various downloads available, worksheets, podcasts and videos.

Finally, we would like to thank you very much for purchasing our book and for the trust you have placed in us.

We wish you all the best, much joy, and energy for your future. Above all, however, we wish you good health, accompanying your diabetes!

Many greetings

Ashley, Emily, and Vivi

Key Words/Directory

Honeymoon Phase: A temporary remission of disease symptoms shortly after the onset of insulin therapy for type 1 diabetes.

Insulin resistance: The body can no longer absorb insulin to metabolise and break down the sugar. This increases the blood sugar level.

BMI = Body-Mass-Index. It is a measure of the evaluation of a person's body weight in relation to his or her height.

Hypos = Abreviations for hypoglycemia = low sugar

Fast acting carbohydrates go quickly into the blood because they are less rich in fibre, e.g. glucose or fruit juice.

Symptoms of type 1 diabetes: Wort & Bild Verlag Konradshöhe GmbH & Co. KG, Apotheken Umschau: Diabetes Ratgeber.

VdK Deutschland e.V.: Application for the severely handicapped pass: Sozialverband.

Type 1 Diabetes during Pregnancy. www.babyundfamilie.de.

German Disability pass explanation: A lump sum is a minimum amount which is credited without having to prove individual amounts, e.g. by means of supporting documents.

RESOURCES

Table 1- Overview of Blood Sugar Levels:

"Diagnosis." *ADA*, American Diabetes Association, www.diabetes.org/diabetes-basics/diagnosis/.

Table 2- Target Values for Diabetics Chart:

"The Big Picture: Checking Your Blood Glucose." *ADA*, American Diabetes Association, www.diabetes.org/living-with-diabetes/treatment-and-care/blood-glucose-control/checking-your-blood-glucose.html.

Table 3- Conversion Table for Blood Sugar Values

"Conversion Table for Blood Glucose Monitoring." *Joslin Diabetes Center*. Joslin Diabetes Center, www.joslin.org/info/conversion_table_for_blood_glucose_monitoring.html.

Typical Symptoms of Type 1 Diabetes:

"Symptoms." *JDRF*, Juvenile Diabetes Research Foundation, www.jdrf.org/t1d-resources/about/symptoms/.

Disability Card Benefits and Experiences:

"Disability Benefits in Germany." *Angloinfo*, Angloinfo Germany, www.angloinfo.com/how-to/germany/healthcare/people-with-disabilities/disability-benefits.

Hof, Patrick. "Offensive Thinking." *Disability Passes in Germany*, Offensive Thinking, 16 Mar. 2014, bt.offensivethinking.org/blog/2014/03/16/disability-passes-in-germany.html.

Severely Disabled Pass Tax-Saving Table:

"Behinderung > Steuervorteile." *Behinderung-Steuervorteile: "Disability: Tax Benefits"*, Betanet. Beta Institute Non-Profit, www.betanet.de/behinderung-steuervorteile.html

Other Sources:

American Diabetes Association, *ADA*, www.diabetes.org/.

Penketh, Anne, et al. "Which Are the Best Countries in the World to Live in If You Are Unemployed or Disabled?" *The Guardian*, Guardian News and Media, 15 Apr. 2015, www.theguardian.com/politics/2015/apr/15/which-best-countries-live-unemployed-disabled-benefits.

Köbsell, Swantje. "The Disability Rights Movement in Germany: History, Development, Present State." *Owards Self-Determination and Equalization: A Short History of the German Disability Rights Movement*, Disability Studies Quarterly, 2006, dsq-sds.org/article/view/692/869.

www.ingramcontent.com/pod-product-compliance
Lightning Source LLC
Chambersburg PA
CBHW072027230526
45466CB00020B/1024